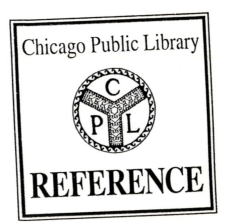

Chicago Public Library

REFERENCE

Form 178 rev. 1-94

FORM 19

IS MENSTRUATION OBSOLETE?

Is Menstruation Obsolete?

by
Elsimar M. Coutinho, M.D., Ph.D.
with
Sheldon J. Segal, Ph.D., M.D. (h.c.),
FRCOG

New York   Oxford
OXFORD UNIVERSITY PRESS
1999

Oxford University Press

Oxford   New York

Athens   Auckland   Bangkok   Bogotá   Buenos Aires   Calcutta
Cape Town   Chennai   Dar es Salaam   Delhi   Florence   Hong Kong   Istanbul
Karachi   Kuala Lumpur   Madrid   Melbourne   Mexico City   Mumbai
Nairobi   Paris   São Paulo   Singapore   Taipei   Tokyo   Toronto   Warsaw

and associated companies in

Berlin   Ibadan

Published by Oxford University Press, Inc.
198 Madison Avenue, New York, New York 10016

Oxford is a registered trademark of Oxford University Press

Library of Congress Cataloging-in-Publication Data
Coutinho, Elsimar M.
Is menstruation obsolete? / by Elsimar M. Coutinho, with
Sheldon J. Segal.
p. cm.
Includes bibliographical references and index.
ISBN 0-19-513021-9
1. Menstruation disorders.   2. Menstruation—Social aspects.
3. Generative organs, Female—Diseases.   4. Women—Health and
hygiene.   I. Segal, Sheldon J.   II. Title.
RG161.C67 1999 618.1'72—dc21 99-17765

1 3 5 7 9 8 6 4 2

Printed in the United States of America
on acid-free paper

*THIS BOOK IS DEDICATED
TO MY LOVING COMPANION TERESA*

*The advice offered in this book is based on the author's experience
with many patients in over thirty years of practice.
It is not, however, intended to be a substitute
for the advice and recommendations
of the reader's personal
physician.*

Contents

Acknowledgments

I would like to convey my gratitude to the following people for their participation in the preparation of this book:

- Sheldon Segal for believing right from the beginning in the concept that menstruation suppression is beneficial, for agreeing to take on the task of getting the book published in the U.S., and for transforming the original manuscript into a book suitable for the U.S. market;

- Lesley Hanson de Moura, my assistant, for her help and competence in the translation of this book from Portuguese into English;

- Kirk Jensen, my editor, for his enthusiasm on reading the manuscript for the first time and for his constant encouragement and helpful comments throughout the process;

- Harriet Segal for her helpful comments, interest, and enthusiasm at every stage of the rewriting of the manuscript;

- Susan Fensten, my publicist, for using her talent to ensure the success of the final product.

SALVADOR, BAHIA, BRAZIL   ELSIMAR M. COUTINHO

Foreword

Menstruation is powerful. Throughout history and without exception, all societies have assigned it some special meaning: mystery, pollution, rite, symbol, secret, or threat. The menstruating woman has been treated in distinct and often rigidly prescribed ways and both women and men together have historically enforced these taboos. Clearly, something about this mysterious monthly discharge of the uterine lining affects us deeply. The history of menstrual beliefs and attitudes is rich, and its legacy leaves some contemporary women with a particular attachment to their menses. These beliefs are part of our shared experience, and are meaningful in their own right.

But they are not necessarily meaningful medically. As this book will argue, regular monthly menstruation is not the "natural" state of women, and it actually places women at risk for several medical conditions of varying severity. Moreover, suppressing menstruation, particularly by continuous oral contraceptive use or other hormonal methods, has remarkable health advantages. In short, the cultural value of menstruation is simply not related to its physiological value.

This message will no doubt be interpreted politically. Especially in the 1970s and 1980s women in the United States reacted against the "medicalization" and "pathologization" of menstruation by physicians and advertisers. Women had been given the consistent message that menstruation is not only shameful and messy, but also is to be concealed from sexual partners and families at all costs. These messages are still very much existent in the popular culture today. For the most part, menstruation is not to be discussed in social or work environments, advertisements for menstrual products emphasize discreetness, and PMS sufferers are expected largely to medicate or remove themselves for fear of giving offense to others.

These messages do exist, but women certainly also have the capacity to think clearly about novel information regarding menstruation. *Is Menstruation Obsolete?* argues for menstrual suppression based on improving women's medical health. The discussion does *not* involve wresting control of women's bodies in order to place it in the hands of doctors, nor exhortations to conceal evidence of menstruation, nor attempts to suppress or erase women's femininity. Instead, it presents a fresh view of menstruation, ultimately concluding that regular menstruation over the course of a woman's reproductive years is simply not necessary from a medical perspective. It is then up to the reader to decide whether these arguments outweigh her personal feelings about menstruation.

Chapters four and five catalog the medical difficulties that can arise from regular menstruation, and chapter seven presents the risks of various forms of medical suppression of menstruation. The reader is encouraged to follow along this direct comparison of two paths, regular menstruation or menstrual suppression, and consider it with a fresh eye. This is not a comparison of a "natural" path with an "artificial" one, but rather a characterization of two long-term physical states with different ramifications for health and daily life.

One of the difficulties of regular menstruation is the usual assembly of monthly symptoms—cramps, headache, fatigue, irritability—which are often dismissed as a part of "the curse" that women must simply endure. Since women tolerate these symptoms so regularly, they may not automatically include them in the "risks" of monthly menstruation. Again, the reader is encouraged to recognize what may have previously gone unnoticed: that this monthly discomfort is simply not obligatory. In fact, it can be a startling exercise for a woman to imagine her life without the hassles and ailments of regular menstruation.

This is a message whose time has come. Fifty years ago women and men lived with certain immutable assumptions about the reproductive process: that human eggs could not be fertilized outside the body, that a woman's pregnancy must involve her own egg, that an anovulatory woman could never conceive, etc. By now, these medical barriers have all been broken, and their use by individuals and couples have found gradual acceptance in society. This book's conception of menstruation is perhaps another example of the medically "immutable" rendered healthfully under the control of individual women.

PHILADELPHIA, PA

KATE MILLER, M.P.H.
UNIVERSITY OF PENNSYLVANIA

Preface

The Portuguese edition of this book was published in 1996 under the title *Menstruação, a Sangria Inútil (Menstruation, a Useless Bleeding)*. As this title implies, Elsimar Coutinho's take-home message for his readers was that from a medical point of view, menstruation has no beneficial effects for anyone, and for many women it is harmful to their health. He also explained how menstruation can be controlled by natural means or by medical intervention and described his experience with the acceptability to women of menstruation suppression, based on his pioneering work with the injectable progestin, DepoProvera®.

I agreed to work with Dr. Coutinho on creating an English-language edition because I believed that American women could benefit from a frank and open discussion regarding the effects of menstruation on women's health.

The reception the book received in Brazil illustrates, not surprisingly, that the subject is highly emotionally charged. Some women interpreted the book as an attack on menstruation and resented the implication that there was something inherently wrong with a process so fundamentally feminine as the monthly periods. Their view was that which is natural has to be beneficial, and that "over-medicalizing" the issue was a failure to recognize the cultural, social, and psychological aspects of what menstruation means to women. Others, particularly those who had personally experienced menstrual cycle–related disorders, were angered to learn that they had never been informed previously of being able to control the monthly anguish they had lived with for most of their adult lives. Many women had heard about the possibility to use hormones, usually birth control pills or injections, to postpone menstruation and were pleased to have an opportunity to learn more about the subject in greater detail.

During my frequent visits to Brazil, I was amazed to observe the extent to which Coutinho's book had prompted media and public discussions of so personal a subject as menstruation. Brazil is, after all, a conservative culture on such matters. There were few women's magazines or television talk shows in the country that didn't do a story on the subject. Usually, Coutinho was invited to discuss his book along with another physician who held the traditional view about suppressing menstruation, or with a skeptical feminist spokeswoman.

The association of frequent menstruation with deleterious health effects has been discussed in the medical literature for many years. Titles such as *Early Menarche, a Risk Factor for Breast Cancer, Indicates Early Onset of Ovulatory Cycles,* or *Incessant Ovulation—a Factor in Ovarian Neoplasia* can be found in respected medical journals as early as 1971. It has also not escaped scientific attention over the years that modern woman, endowed with essentially the same gene pool as her Stone Age ancestors, has a totally different reproductive pattern. Many scientific publications have discussed the fact that over the millennia, women have moved from the age of incessant reproduction to the age of incessant menstruation. If the entire historical presence of womankind on earth were to be represented as a twenty-four-hour day, the time that women have had regular menstrual cycles as the normal pattern of their reproductive years would be just a few seconds of the recent past. Menstruation's emergence as a regular part of life for modern women is the result of cultural changes, drastic reduction of the fertility rate, and a shortening of the duration of breastfeeding, first in the industrialized countries of the West, and more recently in the world's poorer countries.

In this relatively short phase of women's history, menstruation has come to symbolize many important personal attributes: coming of age as a woman, the ability to have children, femininity, and the vigor of youthfulness as opposed to the aging phase of life characterized by menopause. These are important to each woman's self-image as well as to how she is perceived by those around her. In some cultures a potential bride who does not menstruate regularly is considered unlikely to conceive easily and carries a badge of undesirability.

Classical paradigms of medicine are not easy to change. The image of menstruation as natural, normal, and beneficial can be traced back to Hippocrates, the father of medicine, at a time when the Age of Reason began to supplant mythology, but when practitioners of medicine were still naïve about human physiology. With Coutinho, I agree that the time has come to assess menstruation's effects on the health of women from the perspective of modern biology and medicine.

Is Menstruation Obsolete? is a revision of Elsimar Coutinho's original book. In preparing the manuscript for an American audience, we have benefited from the help and advice of many colleagues. Kate Miller, M.P.H., of the University of Pennsylvania, read every chapter and offered a woman's point of view as well as a social scientist's critique on both the factual material included and information omitted, and brought to our attention many new references. She also graciously agreed to write the insightful Foreword to this edition. Andrew Blum, M.D., Ph.D., of Harvard Medical School, reviewed the section pertaining to menstrual cycle–related disorders, particularly concerning epilepsy and migraines, areas of his particular expertise. Michael Miyamoto, Ph.D., of the University of Florida, provided insights, information, and references essential for the discussion of comparative evolution and primatology. Sharon Golub, Ph.D., sent a copy of her excellent book, *Periods: From Menarche to Menopause,* which helped considerably in my understanding of a woman's perspective and in finding and checking important references. Joan Haldenstein, Ph.D., a Greek classicist, kindly provided me with a copy of *Porneia: On Desire and the Body in Antiquity*, by Aline Rousselle, an invaluable reference source on attitudes toward sexual matters in antiquity. Luigi Mastroianni, Jr., M.D., Professor of Obstetrics and Gynecology at the University of Pennsylvania, was constantly available to answer my queries about clinical matters pertaining to gynecology in general and to menstruation-related issues. To all of these colleagues and friends I extend my sincere thanks for helping us to avoid errors of commission or omission. Any that have remained, however, are our responsibility.

Kirk Jensen, Executive Editor at Oxford University Press, recognized the importance of bringing out an edition of this book for an English-speaking audience and has been of constant assistance in advising on structure, style, and context.

Finally, I wish to express my appreciation to the Rockefeller Foundation for the privilege of a residency at its beautiful Study and Conference Center, Villa Serbelloni in Bellagio, Italy, where the hospitable and dedicated staff facilitated my task in bringing this edition of the book to completion.

NEW YORK   S. J. S.

IS MENSTRUATION OBSOLETE?

Introduction

"My mother told me about menstruation on my eleventh birthday. With a reassuring hug, she said that I would soon start to bleed every month for several days at a time. She added that she, herself, had bled ever since she was twelve and that it was nothing to worry about. The bleeding was harmless. Some girls had cramps during the bleeding episodes but this, according to my mother, was perfectly tolerable. There was no point in rejecting the idea of menstruation, as the recurrent bleeding was called, because it was inevitable, she warned. In fact, it even seemed to be good for you because, according to her doctor, it acted as a monthly purge. 'Nature's way of keeping your insides clean.' Besides, it was a sign of becoming a woman."

This account of how she learned about menstruation was related to me by one of my patients who suffered from severe premenstrual tension and who had twice attempted suicide. She told me that when her first "harmless" menstrual period came, together with "tolerable" cramps, she felt deceived, angry, and trapped. I learned over my years of practicing medicine that many women hated "the curse" for the pain it caused them and the helplessness they felt at being unable to prevent or get rid of it. Is menstruation really harmless? Is it inevitable? Is it always tolerable? Could it be considered a monthly purge, as many doctors believed? These questions and my experience with procedures that prevent menstruation prompted me to examine closely the relationship between menstruation and the health and well-being of women.

—Elsimar Coutinho

Contrary to common belief, regular monthly menstruation became part of a woman's life relatively recently in the historical presence of humans on earth. It is a consequence of societal and cultural changes that cause distant evolutionary adaptations to conflict with the best interests for the health of the modern woman. It is reasonable to assume that at the dawn of the human epoch women menstruated rarely or not at all—it would have been extraordinary for a woman to menstruate regularly.

This is because ancestral women were in constant contact with men. From the time of the menarche, perhaps even before their first menstruation, young women were either pregnant or lactating almost continuously. During pregnancy and lactation they would remain free of menstruation (amenorrheic). Even before the suckling baby was weaned, the mother would often become re-impregnated. A new pregnancy and a period of lactation would follow, prolonging the duration of amenorrhea. Release from this repetitive chain of reproductive events would come only with secondary infertility (most likely caused by tubal infection) that would introduce the experience of regular menstruation, or with the unlikely event of reaching menopause. Pregnancy-related mortality rates for early women must have been astronomical. Spontaneous abortion, miscarriage, complicated labor, post-partum infection, and hemorrhage often caused death. Even today, in countries with poor maternal care by modern standards, a woman can have one chance in twenty-five of dying from a pregnancy-related cause.

Menstruation is a rare event in the animal kingdom, even among the many mammalian species that have uterine pregnancies and provide their newborn with mother's milk. Apart from a few (but not all) non-human primates and, curiously, some bats and shrews, the human female is the only menstruating female. This menstruation is a result of evolutionary adaptations that provided survival value and a reproduction advantage for females to repetitively produce and suckle single offspring that could be carried and cared for through the hardships of nomadic existence. This genetic constitution endowed early women with a reproductive system for an era of fertility that was to last for hundreds of thousands of years.

Modern women carry the genes for the same reproductive system, although the pattern of their reproductive lives is totally different from those distant ancestors. For humans and a few related primate species, the evolutionary transition from multiple offspring litters to the single baby born at a stage of development hardy enough to thrive outside of the mother's womb but dependent on mother's milk, warmth, and care, involved a complex pattern of evolutionary adaptations. Genetic mutations affecting the brain, pituitary gland, ovaries, uterus, mammary glands, as well the production of and sensitivity to hormones had to coalesce.

As evolution progressed, hormones that in lower species had other biological functions were used to regulate the evolving system of mammalian reproduction. A hormone, prolactin, that stimulates the brood patch under the dove's breast feathers, or prompts a female newt to seek water before laying her eggs, became the hormone to control milk production in humans. Ancient molecules were put to new uses as the human reproductive process evolved. The vital pregnancy hormone, hCG, that serves as the basis for all human pregnancy tests, has also been found in bacteria and in the gut of a common crab.

Evolution has programmed mammalian species for different types of reproductive behavior. Many are seasonal breeders so that the female's body undergoes the preparations for pregnancy just once a year, when behavioral changes in both males and females make it virtually certain that a pregnancy will be established. Others are reflex ovulators, which cause the female to release an egg and prepare for a pregnancy only after the stimulation of coitus. But the human female produces a mature egg and prepares each month for initiation of pregnancy—fertilizing of an egg in the fallopian tube and nesting of the fertilized egg five days later in the richly vascular uterine lining. If a pregnancy does not start, the outer layer of the uterine lining sloughs off, many blood vessels rupture, and bleeding occurs. Simply put, a human menstrual period is the result of failure to establish pregnancy during the preceding ovarian cycle. If a woman's ovary releases an egg that does not encounter a virile sperm or is fertilized but does not implant securely in the lining of her uterus, a menstruation results. This very early reproductive failure, which is the outcome of nearly 50 percent of all fertilizations, will appear to be an uneventful menstruation.

Ovulation, preceded by the hormonally controlled transformations of the woman's body, did not evolve to be fruitless. When menstruation occurs, it means that the system failed and, for the sake of reproductive efficiency, would have to be repeated the next month, the month after that, and so on, until a successfully nested fertilized egg starts to develop.

In order to prevent rejection of a fertilized egg with its new genetic constitution, it was necessary to include a means to overcome the body's defense mechanisms against a foreign body within the mosaic of human reproductive adaptations. To achieve this, the lining cells of the human uterus, under the stimulus of ovarian hormones, differentiate each month to an advanced point of no return. This is the so-called decidual reaction of the uterine stroma—specialized cells of the lining. This decidual reaction changes the nature of these cells and prevents an inflammatory response directed at the egg as if it were an invading foreign body. Consequently, the implanting fertilized egg is protected from immunological attack and destruction. But decidualized cells cannot revert to their former state. They have proceeded to a point of no return. They either attain the support of the early pregnancy hormones and take part in forming the placenta, or they must die and be sloughed off as part of the menstrual discharge of a non-fertile cycle. This clears the way for the emergence of a new layer of cells that will undergo the same monthly cycle. This is the inevitable by-product of the human ovarian-uterine cycle that each month produces irreversible changes in the lining cells of the uterus.

Over the years, little attention has been given to the possibility that repeated menstruation, a relatively recent experience for women, could be harmful to their health. The era of menstruation began when human social structure and cultural changes broke the relentless pattern of repetitive pregnancies and prolonged periods of lactation. As women reproduced less, they menstruated more often. Presently, fertilization of an egg during a woman's lifetime is a rare event. Of the endowment of about fifty thousand eggs in the ovaries at birth, fewer than five hundred are ovulated, perhaps ten are fertilized, and usually one, two, or three result in a complete pregnancy and delivery. Societal changes have brought women from the era of reproduction to the era of menstruation, and this change is relatively new. As recently as colonial times in America, women had an average of eight children, with long periods of lactation between frequent pregnancies. Relatively speaking, the colonists were menstruation-free compared to their descendent daughters just a few generations later, who average fewer than two children.

Early philosophers, who by 400 B.C. had established the basis of Western thought, analyzed menstruation using the principles of logic and concluded that regular periodic bleeding did no harm to women. Menstruating women, they concluded, were as healthy and normal as non-menstruating pregnant or lactating women. Hippocrates agreed with those philosophers and introduced the concept that menstruation had the function of purging women of bad humors. He did not attempt to address the question of what became of the "bad humors" of men, boys, young girls, or elderly women. This interpretation dominated the attitude of medical doctors regarding menstruation for the following two thousand years. Galen of Rome, the respected follower of Hippocratic teachings, used this doctrine in advocating the use of bloodletting for the treatment of many diseases. In several books he wrote on this subject around 150 B.C. he justified his recommendation by using menstruation as an example of beneficial bleeding, and cruelly attacked anyone who questioned this dogma.

Throughout the ages and up to the beginning of the twentieth century, menstruation-inspired bloodletting was practiced by the greatest of medical authorities. Rooted in tradition and lack of alternatives, doctors routinely bled their patients as a part of established medical procedure. Bloodletting, in fact, caused the death of George Washington, who was bled excessively by the first president's physicians in an effort to treat him for injuries and infection sustained in a riding accident.

Dr. William Osler, one of the most influential medical teachers of the twentieth century, used and taught bloodletting as recently as the early 1900s. Among other indications, he prescribed it especially for the treatment of pneumonia, despite his own recognition that most patients treated by this method died. With the discovery of curative drugs, particularly the introduction of antibiotics, and the improvement in diagnostic techniques including the use of X-ray, medicine changed. Bloodletting was practically abandoned and is no longer taught in medical schools. Today's doctors are barely aware of its existence and know little of its history. The practice remains in use only for the treatment of hemochromatosis, a hereditary disease in which iron is deposited in the tissues. In this case, reduction of blood volume and iron stores has scientific validity. Although therapeutic bloodletting has died out, the rationale on which it was based, that women bleed regularly to rid the body of toxins, lives on.

With the arrival of the oral contraceptive pill forty years ago, women had the opportunity to stop menstruating whenever they wanted for the first time in history. This was not, however, how "the pill" was introduced and explained for use by women. Instead, its inventors and the pharmaceutical industry sought to develop a schedule of administration that would permit users to retain a bleeding pattern similar to menstruation. It was the assumption of marketing experts that women would prefer a method that mimicked the monthly cycle, including a pseudomenstruation. They felt that the idea of avoiding menstruation at will was so new that women would be reluctant to accept this radical change from the ideas they grew up with. Thus was created the familiar schedule of pill taking—three weeks on, one week off—so that withdrawal of the pill's hormones would cause a menstrual-like uterine bleeding.

In the early days of the pill's use, the possibility of marketing the pill to allow a woman to maintain a non-bleeding state for several months was proposed by some scientists but never pursued seriously. In the absence of menstruation, it was argued, women would have constant anxiety that they were pregnant and would soon abandon the use of the pill as a contraceptive. This was before the advent of do-it-yourself pregnancy kits available at the supermarket or local pharmacy. The idea of not allowing the uterine lining to break down and bleed regularly was also resisted by some pathologists who feared this could contribute to the development of endometrial cancer. This argument failed to differentiate between the inner layer of the uterine lining where neoplastic cells emerge, which is not disrupted during menstruation, from the outer layer, that is shed during a menstrual flow.

At that time, there was no marketing effort to test women's acceptability to reducing the number of bleeding episodes, even though this was possible with the continuous use of contraceptive pills. In fact, the knowledge that women could remain free of menstruation safely as long as they took the pill continuously was not routinely explained to pill users. If asked, individual doctors could accommodate their patients requests by explaining that an untimely bleeding could be avoided for a honeymoon or a vacation trip, for example, or to participate in a sporting event, simply by continuing to take the pill without interruption. The pill was packaged in calendar-based dial-packets, in strips with one week of sugar pills, or in packaging with vitamin or iron tablets during the "off week." But never in packages with explanatory labeling to make it convenient for a woman to use the pill to avoid bleeding if she so desired.

In 1959, I was a guest investigator in the laboratory of Dr. George Corner at the Rockefeller Institute for Medical Research (later renamed the Rockefeller University) in New York City. Dr. Corner was a co-discoverer of the hormone he had named progesterone. The word is constructed to describe its function: It *pro*tects *gest*ation and is a *ster*oid hormone. Credit for discovering progesterone is shared between Corner, an anatomist, and Willard Allen, an obstetrician and gynecologist. At the Rockefeller Institute, I met Dr. Sheldon Segal, an endocrinologist, who directed a laboratory research program studying the mechanism of action of hormones and carrying out research on new methods of contraception. The subject of my work was progesterone and how it suppresses ovulation, uterine contractions, and menstruation during pregnancy. If this did not happen, a human pregnancy could not survive. According to prevailing theory, progesterone was responsible for what was called the "progesterone block" which prevented the uterus from contracting during pregnancy. My association with Dr. Segal introduced me to the importance of research on contraception. Women had few choices they could depend on, and the acceptance of the new pill was an uncertainty.

Before returning to Brazil, I learned about medroxyprogesterone acetate (MPA), a new progesterone derivative synthesized by chemists at the Upjohn pharmaceutical company of Kalamazoo, Michigan. MPA was many times more potent than the natural hormone itself and had a prolonged, progesterone-like effect in women. The United States Food and Drug Administration had cleared the new drug, named DepoProvera®, for clinical trials to prevent late-term spontaneous abortion and premature delivery. It was a time when the country was saddened by first lady Jacqueline

Kennedy's loss of a near-term pregnancy because of premature delivery that her physicians were unable to prevent. The use of progesterone to prevent threatened spontaneous abortion or to block premature delivery was based on the hypothesis that the underlying problem in these cases was progesterone deficiency.

Returning to Brazil, I undertook a clinical trial with DepoProvera®, but the treatment failed to prevent either spontaneous abortion or premature delivery. Volunteers participating in these trials had not been deprived of other acceptable treatment. At that time, to preserve pregnancies in women with a history of habitual abortion or premature delivery, bed rest was the only intervention available. In our study, by the scheduled six-month follow-up visit after stopping DepoProvera® treatment, to our surprise, none of the women had resumed ovulating. Therefore, they had not menstruated during the half year. Soon after the six-month check-up, however, the women started to ovulate and become pregnant again.

The study serendipitously led to the discovery of the first long-acting injectable contraceptive. My group at the University Hospital in Bahia, Brazil proved that DepoProvera® could prevent ovulation and menstruation for six months. In a series of clinical trials involving volunteers who did not want to conceive, we learned that ovulation and menstruation could be inhibited for one, three, or six months, depending on the dose of MPA. When I conveyed these results to Upjohn company officials, they were as surprised as I had been, but approval for continuing my studies came directly from the president of the company after a visit to Brazil, and I was provided with the necessary supply of MPA.

Our work with DepoProvera® enabled me to learn firsthand the effect of menstruation suppression for various time intervals. Women who suffered from premenstrual tension and other menstrual disorders welcomed the long menstruation-free intervals. Those with anemia had their iron stores replenished and their blood levels of hemoglobin raised during the period of menstruation suppression. It was clear that, contrary to conventional wisdom, women not only accepted the idea of not menstruating, they appreciated it as a benefit of the treatment.

Similar results were achieved with the uninterrupted administration of oral contraceptives for periods of two, three, six, or twelve months at a time. Women were able to induce withdrawal bleeding whenever they wished by stopping the pill. The idea that women could choose not to menstruate sparked a controversy among medical colleagues. Some feared that menstruation suppression could be harmful. The reaction from the more conservative members of the medical establishment was extreme, criticizing the studies severely and claiming that the inhibition of menstruation was tantamount to transforming women into men. In fact, one group demanded that the police chief of Salvador investigate my research. The dean of the medical school in Bahia responded by requesting the expert opinion of the prestigious Endocrine Society of Brazil, which declared the allegations baseless and the matter was dropped.

Now, over thirty-five years later, DepoProvera® is in wide use. After a thorough study, the World Health Organization endorsed DepoProvera® for long-term use, declaring it safe and effective as a contraceptive. The drug has now been approved all over the world. In the United States (one of the last countries to approve DepoProvera®'s use) its popularity has grown since becoming available for contraception in 1992. I could not have known nearly forty years earlier that by 1998 DepoProvera®, at exactly the same dose and schedule we studied, would be credited for bringing about a dramatic reduction in unwanted teenage pregnancies in the United States. Worldwide, more than ten million women now use DepoProvera® for contraception. They each have the added benefits of long periods free from menstruation. For many women bordering on anemia, this means a return to their normal iron stores and an improvement in overall stamina and resistance to disease.

In addition to DepoProvera®, and as we touched upon earlier, studies have demonstrated that the contraceptive pill can also be used to postpone menstruation. Administered either orally or vaginally, the contraceptive pills can be taken continuously, with only occasional interruption according to the user's wishes. The majority of pill-users and many health care providers are not fully informed of this possibility and its advantages for the prevention of premenstrual syndrome, dysmenorrhea, and other often troubling medical conditions associated with menstruation. Premenstrual syndrome is a cyclical disorder characterized by mood changes and uncomfortable physical symptoms that can occur for many women as the menstrual period approaches. It disappears at or soon after the beginning of menstruation. For many women, these periodic symptoms are sufficiently serious enough to interfere with their work and social life. Myomas and endometriosis are two major causes of physical suffering for many women. Myomas are benign fibroid tumors of the muscular layer of the uterus. Endometriosis is a disease that causes extreme abdominal pain during menstruation and usually is caused by the reflux of menstrual blood and cells discharged through the fallopian tubes into the pelvic cavity. The disease is becoming more common in all countries, as women reach the menarche at an earlier age and menstruate more frequently due to fewer pregnancies and shorter periods of breast feeding. In addition to abdominal pain during menstruation, women with endometriosis can also experience pain associated with intercourse and difficulty in conceiving or maintaining a pregnancy. Unlike endometriosis, myomas are not caused by menstruation but become dangerous during menstruation because a uterus with a large myoma can bleed excessively.

Some women who develop endometriosis have no other choice but surgery, which frequently means permanent loss of fertility. Conservative treatment in less severe cases is based on the administration of a drug that can block the growth-stimulating effects of estrogens and progesterone on the uterus. The most extensively used drug for this purpose is a hormone-like steroid called Danazol®, but its side effects and high cost limit its utility. Another steroid hormone with anti-estrogenic activity, synthesized by a French pharmaceutical firm, is also effective for endometriosis. Named Gestrinone®, the drug inhibits the growth of both the muscular layer and the internal lining of the uterus, causing a reversible uterine atrophy. Our team of Brazilian researchers in Bahia developed this treatment for endometriosis and myomas. Again it is based mainly on suppression of ovulation and menstruation. Taken orally every other day, Gestrinone® is used in several countries and has enabled women with these debilitating conditions to lead pain-free lives. For many, the hope of successful childbearing has also been restored.

The World Health Organization undertook a study in 1983 in ten countries (Egypt, India, Indonesia, Jamaica, Mexico, Pakistan, the Philippines, Korea, United Kingdom, and Yugoslavia) to learn how women feel about menstruation. When asked a series of questions regarding the effects of menstruation on their lives, the majority of respondents of all cultures related some physical discomfort linked to the days preceding bleeding and/or the bleeding days. The most common symptoms were back pain, abdominal pain or bloating, headache, discomfort from breast swelling, and pain in the limbs. Women of all cultures also reported mood changes, although in general, these complaints were less frequent than the physical problems. The conditions most commonly referred to were irritability, lethargy, and depression. The study revealed that lethargy or fatigue was more common in women from developing countries than in those of the more developed countries, probably because of undernourishment and anemia. In every country the majority of women believed that sexual intercourse should be avoided during menstruation.

Despite the many negative aspects of menstruation, amplified in some cultures by taboos which consider menstruating women unclean while excluding them from household, religious, or community functions, the majority of those interviewed did not wish to use a contraceptive method that would suppress menstruation. The reasons for this apparent paradox are complex and understandable. In all cultures, the social constructs around menstruation are strong and have a long history. The widespread beliefs still exist that menstruation is both a natural phenomenon, therefore inevitable, and that any change in its regularity would bring adverse consequences for the woman's health. Many women still view menstruation as a purifying mechanism that rids them of contaminated or bad blood. Similarly, many women also associate menstruation with femininity, fertility, and youth, while considering the end of menstruation with aging and menopause.

Is Menstruation Obsolete? questions some of these widely held beliefs while presenting an alternative perspective on menstruation, particularly for women who experience severe physical or mental suffering during their periodic bleeding.

1

∞

Menstruation in Western Civilization

Menstruation at the Dawn of Civilization

For the hundreds of thousands of years of the prehistoric epoch, with life based on hunting and gathering, the role of women was perceived as producing a child, preferably a man-child. The status of human females began to change when people moved into collective groups, taking up agriculture and abandoning nomadic life. The beginning of agriculture permitted the development of villages, towns, and cities. Social organization began, with tasks and roles allotted to men and women. Agriculture started around eight thousand years before Christ in the plateaus of the Middle East and later extended to the valleys and riverbanks of that region. People abandoned nomadic existence in exchange for a more stable life.

Western civilization is believed to have begun in Sumer and other nearby settlements of southernmost Mesopotamia, between the Tigris and Euphrates rivers, around three thousand five hundred years before the common era (B.C.). People came together in one area, shared their skills and knowledge, and began urban life. From primitive writings in Mesopotamia, modern man has acquired knowledge of the history of the Sumerians, the Babylonians, and the Syrians. The thousands of documents left as clay tablets by the writers of that distant age make it possible to imagine today the lives of those early ancestors at the dawn of civilization.

Under the ruling Syrians, over three thousand years B.C., decrees governing mating were established and marriage was introduced as an official recognition of a union of woman and man. Considering the high mortality of the time because of epidemics and violent wars, childbearing was a goal of great social consequence. The youth who did not marry and have children was criticized, as was the young girl who remained a virgin and did not become pregnant.

Marriages were arranged by parents when the future bride and groom were still children, or sometimes even before they were born. When a young girl reached puberty, she would leave her family and live with the family of her husband, where she would remain until her death. If she did not conceive she could be returned to her family or treated even more harshly. Encouraged by community leaders and aware of the high rate of child mortality, women married in this way would have successive pregnancies, menstruating only rarely. Only those who could not have children experienced menstruating regularly for many years. Rejected by their husbands and stigmatized by the community, many had no choice but to turn to prostitution. The study of hundreds of thousands of documents describing more than three thousand years of civilization in Mesopotamia reveals this pattern of marriage, childbearing, and the relationship between childlessness and prostitution. While these documents hold no specific references to menstruation, we can surmise its rarity in women other than the childless. Since pregnancy and lactation were associated with amenorrhea and not having children meant menstruating, it can be concluded that menstruating regularly was undesirable.

The Persians, who followed the Syrians, considered menstruation as acceptable when it lasted no more than four days. During this period, the women of the family were isolated in special rooms. At the end of four days, if a woman continued bleeding, she would receive one hundred lashes and was put back in isolation for an additional five days. If, after this period of time, she continued to menstruate, she would receive four hundred lashes because "without doubt she was possessed by a bad spirit," and in this case a "purification" in the form of whip-lashing was deemed necessary.

Menstruation in Ancient Greece

As Mesopotamia's influence began to wane, and new centers of civilization developed elsewhere in Europe, Northern Africa, and Asia, ancient Greece became a fountain of knowledge in practically every area of learning. It was in the golden age of Greece, around four hundred years B.C., that early notions of biology, physics, chemistry, philosophy, politics, law, and medicine were formed. Extraordinary men established the foundations of modern science. Although they lived over two thousand years ago, their names are remembered even today because their ideas are still useful for understanding nature and the progress of civilization: Pythagoras, Aristotle, Plato, Archimedes, Democritus, Euclid, Socrates, and Hippocrates. The work *Corpus Hippocraticum*, which documents the ideas of the father of medicine and his contemporaries, has influenced the professional behavior of every doctor who lived during the past two thousand years. Medical graduates still take the Hippocratic Oath when they receive their diplomas and swear to practice medicine according to the principles he put forth.

In Hippocrates' time it was thought that a woman's uterus was sub-divided internally, forming numerous compartments and protuberances, and that the interior of the uterus contained tentacles and suckers. The existence of the ovaries and oviducts (tubes) was not known. Since human corpses were not examined, whatever information existed about the anatomy and function of the human uterus was gained through observations of the uteris of animals. Mostly, this was work carried out by the great scientist and philosopher of the time, Aristotle. However, Hippocrates was the first to consider the phenomenon of menstruation and, based on the knowledge available at the time, he concluded that menstruation was beneficial to women. Hippocrates was impressed by the relief afforded by the onset of menstruation to women who periodically suffered from premenstrual headaches, swelling, and nervousness, and, as explained earlier, concluded that the bleeding was nature's way of getting rid of the bad humors that were responsible for these maladies.

Menstruation During the Roman Empire

The Roman Empire dominated as the center of intellectual life from the second century B.C. until the fourth century A.D. During the first century of the Christian era, around 60 A.D., the geographer and naturalist Pliny the Elder wrote his *Natural History*, the first encyclopedia. This monumental work became a widely read and oft-cited reference source. The major opus was divided into thirty-seven books and was finished in the year 77 A.D. In the volume on human biology, Pliny describes menstrual blood as a deadly poison, which contaminates and decomposes urine, destroys the fertility of seeds, kills insects, withers crops, kills flowers, rots fruit, and blunts knives. Pliny also asserts that if menstruation were to coincide with an eclipse of the moon or of the sun, the resulting evils would be irreparable. He warns that when the sun is in full lunar eclipse, sexual intercourse with a menstruating woman can be fatal to a man.

With the decline of ancient Greece and the loss of the Greek texts on which Pliny based his work, *Natural History* became the textbook most used in general education. In Europe during the Middle Ages, many monastic libraries possessed copies of his work. His authority went unchallenged, either because there was no other more reliable source, or because his statements could not be disproved. The first serious criticism of Pliny's work did not appear until 1492. It was only then, fourteen centuries after his death, that Pliny's influence diminished. By the end of the seventeenth century, *Natural History* had been rejected by the most important scientists of the age. Nevertheless, in the nineteenth century, *Natural History* was still considered one of the major literary works of antiquity, although its reputation for scientific information had long faded. Today, the material contained in its thirty-seven volumes remains an important source of facts about the past and is considered a reliable representation of Rome in the first century A.D.

Around the year 180 A.D., Rome was at its peak and its power extended widely over the civilized world. The most influential Roman doctor of that time was Galen (129–199) who, although he had no special background in women's health matters, set about collecting all the information that was available on the subject. He concentrated particularly on the works of Aristotle, Hippocrates and, principally, the Greek doctors Rufus and Soranus of Ephesus, who had accurately described the human uterus for the first time. Soranus was considered the greatest gynecologist of antiquity. In his textbook, he gave the position and size of the uterus and quite accurately described all the female reproductive organs, including the external genitalia. He included the clitoris but did not explain its function. Like others of his time, he recognized that menstruation was necessary for conception but mistakenly believed that immediately after menstruation was the most fertile time. Soranus' work on gynecology did not reflect a fear of amenorrhea. He recognized it as a clearly identified phenomenon occurring among normal, healthy women, such as singers (Soranus' view) and women who engaged in sports a great deal. If they wished to conceive, he advised, they could do so by changing their lifestyle.

Galen was the first to recognize that the oviducts, later named for the sixteenth century Italian anatomist Fallopius, convey the ova, which he considered to be female sperm, to the uterus. He demonstrated that the vessels carrying menstrual blood to the uterus end in crypts. Despite Galen's major contributions to medicine, some authors are critical of the blind acceptance of his teachings. They believe that this contributed to delaying the progress of medicine for fifteen hundred years.

In the thousand years that followed Galen's death—during the Middle Ages, the Age of Darkness—virtually nothing new was added to medicine. Strange ideas arising from imagination, speculation, and superstition, rather than from observation, were proposed in this period. For example, the idea supported by Galen, that the uterus had various compartments, was embellished with the notion that a male conceptus would develop in the three compartments on the right side, a female conceptus on the left side, and hermaphrodites in the middle compartment.

Although the demographic history of antiquity is uncertain, it is believed that five or six million people lived in Roman Italy at the time of Galen. Along with the free citizens, about two million slaves worked for their masters, either in agriculture or as domestic servants. Since slaves were forbidden to marry, sexual relations among them tended to be promiscuous. Exceptions were those who made hidden vows of fidelity to each other, and male slaves in the service of the Emperor who had the privilege of receiving an exclusive female companion. Although the right to determine who could marry and who could not marry was controlled by the government, Roman marriages were private acts with no formal recognition either from public authorities or religious bodies. Marriage was a verbal agreement between a free man and a free woman who would then live together and constitute a family. The arrangement, however, did establish certain rights for the children of the couple as well as for the widow or widower.

At the beginning of the Christian era, followers of Jesus adopted the concept of monogamy and incorporated it into the new religion's dogma. At that time, the concept of one man, one wife was recent in the emerging Western civilization. When followed, monogamy could serve to preserve a family lineage. The public's acceptance of this objective was probably the basis for the custom of leverate, requiring that a man must take his brother's widow as his wife, incorporated in early Judaism over twenty-five hundred years B.C. The Old Testament describes the story of Onan. When his brother died, Onan married his brother's wife, as custom required, but rather than impregnate her, "he spilled his seed upon the ground." In so doing, Onan practiced a form of contraception that subsequently became the most frequently used method throughout the world. In the modern world, there is a slang expression for the practice of *coitus interruptus* in virtually every language or dialect. In ancient times it was the woman who initiated withdrawal by moving her body away from the man, according to Aline Rousselle in her fine book, *Porneia: On Desire and the Body in Antiquity*.

A Roman proverb of the time of Galen stated, "*A good man should only make love to have children; the state of marriage does not serve venereal pleasures.*" The disciples of Jesus adopted this view and, from the time of its formation, the Catholic Church has maintained the principle of this proverb, derived from pagan Rome, as a strict religious dogma. At the time of the Emperor Augustus, shortly before the birth of Christ, special laws were created to persuade Roman citizens to get married. In their book *Histoire de la Vie Privée*, Aries and Duby propose that monogamous marriage became acceptable when the public began to question why a man and woman should spend their life together solely for the purpose of childbearing and no longer accepted this as an indisputable, natural way of life.

When monogamous marriage became an institution enforced by law, the practice of abortion and contraception, already known in early civilizations, permitted couples to limit the number of children. This also enabled unmarried women and prostitutes to avoid the birth of children. Plato and Cicero refer to the custom of douching after the sexual act. The law permitted this privilege to mothers of three children, since it was considered that women with this number of children had already fulfilled their civic duty. Not everyone ended at three. This may have been partly because of the notorious unreliability of the douching method. Marcus Aurelius (121–180 A.D.) had nine children. Cornelia, considered a model wife, mother of Gracchi, had twelve children.

Menstruation was part of life for those women who remained unmarried. The gynecologist Soranus, without understanding the physiology of reproduction, prescribed that married women should try to conceive immediately before or immediately following menstruation. Recognizing the problems women encountered with menstruation, he counseled virgins, such as the religious Vestal virgins, that, despite "the menstrual difficulties," virginity did not cause any adverse consequences to health. Later, in the second century A.D., Greek philosophers from Stoa developed the Stoic philosophy in which passion, sexual pleasures, contraception, and abortion were condemned. As the influence of Christianity in civilization rose by the third century A.D., the Catholic Church maintained its early embrace of the Stoic attitude towards sex. Men and women began to deliberately abstain from cohabiting, sometimes for their entire earthly life, in the hope of securing their place in heaven. Even for those who did marry, sex was limited to procreation, with the feeling that "God's penetrating eye is everywhere." Celibacy meant that women would menstruate throughout the entire span of their reproductive years.

Menstruation in the Byzantine Middle Ages

Following the occupation of the Roman Empire's western provinces by the Barbarians from the north and Asia, the Greco-Roman world in the West declined. A new age began when "the men of Caesar and Pompey became John, Peter and Matthew," in the words of Niccolo Machiavelli (1469–1527). The influence of the Romans, however, continued for many centuries. In the fifth century, in the "darkness of the High Middle Ages," religion took a keen interest in the private life of individuals. More people lived in the countryside than the city. At that time, the infant mortality rate remained high, around four hundred and fifty per one thousand births. Birth rates and death rates were roughly equal so that there was very little natural population growth. Average lifespan was around forty-five years for men and just thirty-five years for women, who often died at a young age as a result of childbirth or abortion. A man needed to have many wives and many children to ensure survival and continuity of his family. The elderly were rare, but for those who managed to reach forty years of age, the chances of continuing survival increased substantially.

In the year 330 A.D. Constantine, the first Christian Emperor of the Roman Empire, moved his capital from Rome to the ancient Greek city of Byzantium (later named Constantinople and then renamed Istanbul by the Turks). Constantine's conversion to Christianity gave greater power to the Catholic Church, which remained an important influence on the State for centuries. By the end of the fourth century, Rome had gone into decline while Constantinople, the eastern capital, grew in wealth and strength.

Constantine granted the religious authorities the power to create laws establishing the rules of behavior. Hence, the Church controlled the laws regulating relationships between men and women, previously a privilege of the State. The fall of Constantinople to the Turkish Muslims in 1453 marked the end of the Roman Empire in the East and in Asia Minor. This was a severe setback for Christianity. Throughout the Byzantine period, church leaders participated in the administration of civic life and in family and cultural matters. The patriarch answered directly to the emperor, who permitted the Church to occupy the best areas of the city and subsidized the construction of their splendid, rich temples. The Church had begun to exert total control over all human activities, establishing rules concerning how people should dress, eat, walk, and even how they should have sex.

Many restrictions were imposed. Those who chose a monastic life were obliged to renounce sex, dedicate all their physical and mental activity to the service of God, and donate all their material wealth to the Church. The union of two people in marriage acquired a religious character. The works of Sisinios established in 997 that marriage was prohibited between brother and sister, uncles and nieces, nephews and aunts, or first cousins and descendants of first cousins. Formal marriage engagements became important in view of the age limitation for marriage: twelve years for girls and fourteen years for boys. Young women, even if they were not virgins, were obliged to feign virginity. A gynecological manual from that time teaches how to cover up the non-virgin condition by scheduling the wedding night to coincide with the bride's menstrual period. Marriage was the only course for those who were unable to attain "the higher level of virginity or sexual continence," as Paul the Apostle preached.

The use of concubines was officially forbidden by the Church, but was tolerated for those with the means to afford them. Romanus I, father-in-law of Constantine VII and co-emperor, fathered a son by his concubine, as well as a large legitimate family. The child was allowed to survive but was castrated to avoid the formation of a concurrent line of descendants.

Hippocratic and Galenic medicine, including the concept of the four humors (blood, lymph, green bile, and black bile), was taught in medical textbooks. An article on uterine pathology, written by Metrodora between the eleventh and twelfth centuries, attributed an important role to the uterus for the health of women. Serious problems were described for those "who become widowed in the prime of their lives or in virgins who let the right moment for marriage pass them by, leaving the natural desire without use." The book contains cures for illnesses of the uterus and difficulties in conceiving or in giving birth, and teaches how to verify virginity without a physical examination, how to feign virginity, how to provoke orgasm, and even how to confess to adultery.

In the seventh and eighth centuries Islam was transformed into a formal religion, taking on and resolving problems of dogma and theology. The new monotheistic religion, taught by the Prophet Mohammed, rapidly expanded to the Mediterranean region and its followers began to suffer the consequences of Islam's struggle for survival against Christianity, which lasted for many centuries.

The arrival of Islam did little to change medicine in the Middle Ages. However, concern for the Islamic Arab people inspired their rulers to seek in Greek medicine the bases of forming their own remedies. An intensive and extensive translation work, started under the rule of Harun-al Rashid (786–809), was further intensified under the rule of his son Ma'um between 813 and 833. An important milestone in this translation and subsequent incorporation into Arabian culture of important texts from Western learning was the establishment in 832 of the House of Knowledge, Bayt-al-Hikma, in Baghdad. Here, highly competent and dedicated men undertook this enormous task. The most important of these wise men was Hunaym ibn Ishaq, who lived until 873 and later became known in Europe as Johannitius. In one of his works, Hunaym discusses one hundred twenty-nine of Galen's texts that he and his fellow workers translated into Arabian and Syrian.

The era of translations continued up to the eleventh century, and hundreds of texts, including almost all the works of Galen, were translated into Arabic at frenetic speed. Galen was undoubtedly the most translated author, and thus influenced Arabic medical ideas for many centuries. Consequently, his teachings concerning menstruation were adopted in Arabic medicine.

Menstruation in Feudal Europe

At the end of the Middle Ages in feudal Europe the Catholic Church continued to intervene in the conjugal life of married couples, but the church's role became more superficial and ambiguous compared to the power of the feudal lords. At the beginning of the Renaissance, in the fifteenth century, writers expressed distinct doubt about the importance of virginity. However, middle class young women could not have had complete sexual relations before marriage without the inevitable consequence of pregnancy. In fact, *coitus interruptus* was known and practiced at that time. Casual or long-lasting sexual relationships were inevitable, either at home between relatives or servants, or outside the home. The presence of prostitutes in every city was assured by the demand of the enormous number of bachelors who either did not want to or could not take on the responsibility and risks of marriage. In Venice during the sixteenth century, around 1530, there were an estimated eleven thousand prostitutes in the city, a number that reflects the enormous demand. "Daily outings offered opportunities for clandestine meetings and for hearing proposals of furtive encounters."

The fragile morality of the time and the risks resulting from these meetings became a major preoccupation for the Church. Since no notice seemed to be taken of church sermons, steps were taken to intervene. In the fourteenth century, the Dominican and Franciscan monks tried to recoup their influence, visiting families at their dwellings and playing the role of counselors and confidants of those who were not willing to listen to them in church.

The closeness of the monks to the population increased the practice of the confessional and enhanced the control of the Church over the private life of the citizens. The educators and confessors began to compel their pupils and penitents to go through training to enable them to resist the temptations of the senses, "predictors of concupiscence." Concerning sight: "In every part in which sin is found, lower your eyes." With regard to taste, touch, smell, hearing: "Do not hear ... that which you should not." Of course, the training included sexuality for married couples. For unwed people, in principle, sexuality did not exist. Marriage ceremonies could not take place during times prohibited by the Church and it was a mortal sin if the marriage was prematurely consummated. Marriage ceremonies were permitted only in convenient places during certain times. Sodomy was forbidden and considered a very serious, mortal sin, as were unconventional coital positions. The program of the Church demanded the enlistment of hundreds of monks scattered throughout the cities, as well as political and administrative leaders interested in bringing order and civil obedience, which was difficult to obtain without threat of damnation.

During feudal times, the attitude prevailed among the French and the Germans that the essence of marriage is in its consummation and cohabitation. An important gesture was the memento the husband gave to his wife on the morning after the wedding—the *morgengabe* or morning gift—which represented his gratitude to her for remaining a virgin until her wedding day. Virginity was recognized or confirmed, as it still is today, by the occurrence of bleeding during the nuptial relations. Unschooled in human anatomy, particularly regarding the existence of the hymen, husbands based their judgment on the spot of blood discovered on the bed sheets the following morning. Although it was only in the tenth century that virginity became an essential condition for a woman in a first marriage, the husband's gift vouched for the purity of his young wife.

It became necessary in those "troubled times when violence reigned" to protect virgins before marriage because virginity gave an assurance of certainty of paternity, and the marriage and inheritance depended on that certainty. Rape, kidnapping of women, incest, and adultery were considered serious offenses and were harshly punished. The violation of a free woman was punishable by death; of a slave, with the payment of her cost. The value assigned to virginity meant that most women, not only nuns, menstruated regularly. Until they married and became pregnant, all women would have to bleed every month.

Menstruation in the Renaissance

The Renaissance period, when universities and schools of medicine flourished all over the civilized world, began with the fall of Constantinople in 1453. Shortly before, there had already been signs of the end of the Middle Ages. In 1315, for example, the first authorized dissection of a human body for scientific reasons was carried out at the University of Bologna. Nevertheless, it was during the Renaissance, more than a century later, that studies on human anatomy started to be performed systematically, leading to a better understanding of the relationship between organs and the way they work. For example, drawings in books of that period already show the uterus with the appearance it would have if drawn today. However, fantasy was frequently mixed with reality. For example, both Mondino de Luizzi (1275–1290) and Leonardo da Vinci (1452–1519) drew the uterus with veins communicating it with the breast because they believed that menstrual blood was transformed into milk during lactation and for this reason women did not menstruate when they were breast-feeding. Leonardo was the first to draw the ovaries, tubes, and ligaments. During the same period, their contemporary, Berengario da Carpi, stated for the first time that the notion was wrong that the human uterus was sub-divided into compartments.

Andreas Vesalius (1514–1564), a Belgian living in Padua, depicted for the first time in his peerless work, *De Humanis Corporis Fabrica*, the interior of the human body as it really is. Vesalius correctly described the uterus although he still contended that there was a division in its interior. This was not because he had seen any division but to affirm the notion of Galen that there were sub-divisions in the interior of the uterus. The terms *uterus* and *pelvis* were used for the first time in his work. Vesalius's work was continued by some of his disciples. Colombo de Cremona, for example, described and named the vagina and the labia major. He was the first to report a case of congenital absence of the uterus and vagina. Fallopius de Modena provided a detailed description of the tube-like structures leading from the uterus to the region of the ovaries. His name became associated with this anatomical structure, the fallopian tubes, although he denied the priority of discovery attributed to him. Fallopius also described the hymen and the clitoris, as well as the corpus luteum, which is formed by the ovary's vacated follicle after ovulation.

At the same time as the anatomists in Italy were describing details of human anatomy, Englishman William Harvey (1578–1657) discovered the circulation of blood, and the first microscopes were used to begin to see what the naked eye could not see. In 1605, Miguel de Cervantes referred quite naturally to menstruation in his *Don Quixote de la Mancha*, suggesting that at that time the characteristics of menstruation were recognized in a manner similar to today. Concurrently, William Hunter described how the placenta works and demonstrated the existence of the spiral arteries in the endometrium.

Meanwhile, precise information on the microscopic structure of pelvic organs was obtained because of new techniques in preserving and staining of tissues. However, it was only in the eighteenth century that compound microscopes were perfected, making it possible to gain a better understanding of the changes which take place in the endometrium during the menstrual cycle. It was then possible to demonstrate scientifically that the notion of pre-formation was wrong. (This was the long-held view that embryos already existed in the ovary and that pregnancy was merely transferring them to the uterus.)

Menstruation in the Twentieth Century

Despite the progress made in the nineteenth century, scientific evidence that there is normal, cyclical activity in the uterus was not confirmed until the early years of the twentieth century. The classical paper describing the control of changes in the uterus by inner secretions of the ovary was written in 1905 by the Austrian gynecologist Josef Halban. In 1908, Hitschmann and Adler, two German doctors, demonstrated that the alterations in the internal lining of the uterus, the endometrium, interpreted up to that time as pathological, were normal and resulted from the action of Halban's inner secretions (the word *hormone* had not yet been coined). The existence of these ovarian secretions was demonstrated by experiments in which organs were removed from animals and the consequences of their removal observed. The disappearance of specific effects and their re-appearance through the administration of extracts of the removed organ confirmed the existence of the internal secretion. This is the so-called ablation and replacement experiment, a mainstay of endocrinology research even today.

Halban's work showed that the mammalian ovary exerted an influence on the behavior and physiology of animals. This was demonstrated by observing the effects of removing the ovaries. The secretion responsible for these effects, he learned, is produced in greater quantity at regular intervals, causing the condition characterized as pro-estrus and estrus (heat). It was known that during these periods the egg matures and the follicle bursts. After ovulation, the corpus luteum forms and this organ provides another secretion whose function appeared to be essential for the alterations which occur during the implantation and development of the embryo in the first stages of pregnancy.

Robert Schroder (1909) was the first to use the terms *proliferative* and *secretory* to describe the pre- and post-ovulatory phases of the human endometrium and to demonstrate the existence of a basal layer that remains intact and a functional layer that deteriorates during menstruation. Schroder published many papers between 1909 and 1915 on the cyclic alterations of the endometrium and was the first to attribute endometrial hyperplasia, a pathological condition, to the persistent action of secretions from the ovary.

In 1926, Bernhard Zondek and Louis Ascheim demonstrated the presence of estrins in the ovary but the stimulating effect of these estrogenic secretions on the growth and contractility of the human uterus would only be well documented much later. When he was a young doctor in pre–World War II Germany, Zondek also discovered the presence of estrogenic material in the ovary and in the urine of the pregnant mare. After he fled the Nazis and re-settled at Hebrew University in Jerusalem, his continued work led to the development of Premarin®, the hormone replacement therapy most used by American women to overcome the problems of menopause. The influence of the pituitary gland's hormones on the ovary was recognized, thanks to the classic research carried out by Smith and Engle in the United States, and Zondek and Ascheim in Germany.

Progesterone was discovered in 1929 by George Corner and Willard Allen. Its effects on the inhibition of uterine contractility, indispensable for the maintenance of pregnancy, and its participation in the preparation of the endometrium for pregnancy were recognized soon after. In 1931 George Bartelmez demonstrated that an important stage in the shedding of the endometrium during menstruation is the closing of the spiral arteries thus depriving the cells of their oxygen and nutrition.

The discovery of crystalline progesterone in 1934 made possible the detailed investigation of its functions in the human menstrual cycle. Artificial cycles were soon being created in menopausal women, simulating ovulatory menstrual cycles. A perfect menstrual cycle was obtained with the administration of estrogen followed by the administration of progesterone and estrogen. When the administration of the combination of estrogen and progesterone was discontinued, a bleeding of several days' duration began exactly like a menstrual period. And so it was that, through "experimental medicine," the mechanisms responsible for the mysterious bleeding were discovered. In 1940, John Markee carried out an ingenious experiment in *rhesus* monkeys in which he demonstrated the occurrence of menstruation in fragments of endometrium transplanted to the anterior chamber of the eye where daily events could be observed over a prolonged period of time. The vital role of the pregnancy hormone, human chorionic gonadotropin (hCG) was finally demonstrated in women in the 1950s.

Despite the avalanche of information which revealed the benign character of menstruation, some scientists still persisted with the erroneous concepts regarding menstrual blood, which had existed since the times of Pliny. In 1952, Olive and George Smith of Harvard University, pioneers in the clinical use of estrogen and recognized authorities in gynecology, proposed the theory of the existence of a toxic substance in menstrual blood, menotoxin, the presence of which they had announced some years previously. According to them, laboratory animals injected with menstrual blood invariably died. In Jerusalem, Bernhard Zondek repeated the Smith experiments. However, Zondek added antibiotics when he injected menstrual blood. The antibiotics prevented the death of the animals, thus demonstrating that the lethal effect of the menstrual blood injected into mice by the Smiths was not caused by toxins, but by bacterial infection as a result of the contamination of the menstrual blood by bacteria from the vagina. Although the experiments repeated by Zondek did not confirm their findings, the Smiths continued to hold their opinion concerning "menotoxin" for many years.

Despite the extraordinary progress made in the endocrinology of reproduction in the first half of the twentieth century, nothing compares to the information explosion which took place in the second half.

Up to the 1950s, the hormones which participate in the reproductive cascade—estrogen, androgen, progesterone, and the gonadotropins—were researched and measured in human blood and in urine using complicated and imprecise methods that required the extraction and purification of the hormone in relatively large amounts of blood and urine. There were chemical methods and the so-called bioassays. Human blood or urine samples were injected into a laboratory animal and the effects on the animal's sex organs were examined. The Galli-Manini test, for example, consisted of injecting a woman's urine into a male frog, waiting for a few minutes, and examining the frog's urine under a microscope. The presence of spermatozoa indicated a positive pregnancy test. Human chorionic gonadotropin is produced early in a woman's pregnancy. Its presence in the urine causes the release of sperm in the frog. The active hormone in the familiar rabbit test for pregnancy and the A-Z test in mice is hCG. Now that women can use at-home pregnancy test kits, it is still hCG that they test for by an immunologic reaction on a strip of paper. This is the hormone that stimulates the production of progesterone in pregnant women. It is essential to prevent an ensuing menstruation which would be disastrous for the nascent pregnancy. Acting on the pituitary gland, progesterone indirectly prevents further ovulation for the remainder of the pregnancy. It also is essential for preparing the uterine lining for implantation of a fertilized egg.

Although very sensitive, the biological methods were not reliable because of individual differences in the response of the animals used in the tests. In the 1960s, immunological and radioisotopic methods were introduced, which enabled the identification and measurement of the hormones precisely, quickly, and in much smaller amounts of blood and urine. These methods, which are even simpler today with the use of enzymes, permitted an explosion of knowledge unprecedented in the history of medical endocrinology.

It was only after the appearance of oral contraceptives by 1960 that, for the first time in human history, women were given the option of controlling their own menstrual cycle: prolonging it, shortening it, or simply abolishing it.

2

∝

Menstruation:
The Basis of Therapeutic Bloodletting

Hippocrates of Ancient Greece

When ancient Greece stood as the fountain of medical knowledge in the Western world, menstruation was considered beneficial to women's health. This positive interpretation reflected the opinion of prestigious doctors, influenced by the legendary Hippocrates, the father of medicine. Not understanding why women bled periodically, Hippocrates based his favorable opinion on the observation that the arrival of the menstrual period brought noticeable relief of symptoms for women who suffered severe headaches, nervous tension, and other physical symptoms in the premenstrual days. Unaware of ovulation or even of blood circulation, the founder of observation-based medicine could only interpret the menstrual flow as the natural way to alleviate the monthly distress of many women. He had no way of knowing that the premenstrual days were physiologically a part of the cyclical events that centered around ovulation and terminated with menstruation itself. He reasoned that since neither men nor pregnant women suffered from the periodic mood changes and physical symptoms that affected non-pregnant women, they had no reason to bleed.

A philosopher as well as physician, Hippocrates believed in studying facts and drawing conclusions from observations, in the tradition of his contemporary, Socrates. Hippocrates applied logic and reason to medicine and took it out of the realm of religion and mysticism. His belief in the benefits of menstrual bleeding for women's health led him to endorse bloodletting as a cure for health problems in men similar to those that periodically afflicted women. If menstruation ended a woman's suffering from certain symptoms, men with the same complaints should benefit from an induced blood loss, he reasoned. He prescribed it for men who were emotionally disturbed, nervous, or suffered from headaches. The indications for this treatment gradually became broader through the centuries as medicine acquired more credibility than witchcraft or magic for resolving health problems. From the time of Hippocrates up to the beginning of the twentieth century, bloodletting became a principal tool of medical practitioners to combat acute illness, chronic disease, traumatic injuries, and even devastating epidemics.

Hippocrates interpreted other bouts of blood loss that occurred in either women or men as having beneficial and even curative effects. In his writings, he described the miraculous benefit of spontaneous bleeds in victims of an epidemic that brought fever and paralysis. When individuals afflicted with this mysterious fever bled copiously from the nose, he concluded, they survived. The father of medicine wrote that during the epidemic, none of his patients who had bled "adequately" through the nose, died. He reported that three of his patients had a slight bleeding on the fourth and fifth days of the sickness but did not survive. Hippocrates concluded that the extent of their bleeding was insufficient to save them. The lifesaving hemorrhages benefited especially young persons and those in the prime of life. "Those who had not the hemorrhage (who were obviously the elderly), died," he wrote. Although he made this astute observation, Hippocrates did not attribute the resistance of surviving patients to youthful vigor, but rather to the occurrence of nasal bleeding. He also related menstruation to the progress of the fever. "There were fewer deaths among women than men," he wrote. "Females had the menstrual discharge during the fever, and many girls had it then for the first time; in certain individuals both the hemorrhage from the nose and the menses appeared." He continued, "I knew no instance of any one dying when . . . these took place properly."

Hippocrates described another epidemic that occurred with the weather change of early winter. In those most seriously afflicted, along with fever, other symptoms included: "thirst, nausea, delirious talking, fears, despondency, great coldness of the extremities." These symptoms did not occur, he concluded, when there was a hemorrhage from the nose. He found that when this illness befell women and girls, "whoever of them had abundant menstruation were saved thereby so that I do not know a single female who had any of these favorable [circumstances, i.e. menstrual bleeding] that died."

Based on his conviction that hemorrhages were always beneficial, Hippocrates recommended bleeding patients for whom he had no alternative treatment. This was the majority of afflictions. In treating acute illnesses, he recommended: "Bleed in acute affections, if the disease appears strong, and the patients are in the vigor of life, and if they have strength." In cases of pleurisy, Hippocrates advised an intestinal purge or enema, but bloodletting, he maintained, "holds the first place in conducting the treatment." Bleeding and purging together, he warned, "require caution and moderation."

His recommendations on when and how to apply bloodletting were highly specific. "When a person suddenly loses his speech, in connection with obstruction of the veins, if this happens without warning . . . one ought to open the internal vein of the right arm, and extract blood more or less according to the habit and age of the patient." Hippocrates mentions venesection specifically as a treatment for dysuria (difficult or painful urination) and for pain in the eyes.

Curative bloodletting did not originate with Hippocrates but he reinforced its acceptance in curative medicine. His birth in ancient Greece is believed to have been around the year 460 B.C. Some biographers describe him as a descendent of the god Asclepius (Aesculapius, in the Roman spelling). In Greek mythology, it was not unusual for mortals, such as Hippocrates, to be associated with divinities; many Greek heroes claimed gods as their ancestors. Asclepius, symbolized in art and sculpture by the serpent-entwined staff, was the god of healing. His staff remains the symbol of medicine today. For centuries, relief from affliction was religiously based on worship in temples of healing built to honor him. According to Greek mythology, the family of Hippocrates descended from a son of Asclepius, who survived the Trojan war (1194–1184 B.C.). Returning from Troy, he saved the life of a princess by performing bloodletting and the grateful king gave the healer his daughter's hand in marriage. They had two sons who continued the tradition of their grandfather and father in practicing the art of healing.

Eventually, one branch of this medical family established itself on the island of Cos, off the coast of Asia Minor. This is where Hippocrates was born many centuries and nineteen generations later. Ignoring the temples of healing dedicated to Asclepius, he practiced and taught medicine as a science based on reason rather than god-worship. His reputation grew and, because of him, tiny Cos became famous throughout the Western world as a medical center. Hippocrates treated his patients on the basis of fact and observation. His theories on medicine are summed up in *Corpus Hippocraticum*, which contains more than seventy treatises on medicine and scientific subjects. Some were written by him; others were added over the years as disciples recorded Hippocratic teachings that were handed down from generation to generation, or by doctors who ascribed to him their pet theories in order to give them greater credence.

Hippocrates championed the principle that the first goal of the physician is the care and cure of the patient. For both his science and philosophy, he achieved the renown and respect that earned him the title "father of medicine." Even today, most young doctors take the Hippocratic Oath when receiving the diploma to practice medicine.

This account of the life of a mortal man, commingled with mythology, reveals that bloodletting may have been carried out many hundreds of years before Hippocrates was born. Even artifacts from ancient Egypt, 2500 B.C., depict venesection, most likely being used as a healing process. Hippocrates legitimized and rationalized the procedure on the observational basis of the presumed benefits of menstruation for the health of women, and on other examples of blood loss that, to him, appeared relevant in the cure of sick people.

Galen, the Prince of Medicine, and the Defense of Bloodletting

The *Corpus Hippocraticum* dominated medicine for many centuries. Practically every doctor in the Western world adopted its ideas and treatments. In the second century B.C. the Roman physician Claudius Galenus became a zealous supporter and defender of Hippocratic teachings. Galen, as he came to be known, himself was destined to become one of the most famous physician/teachers in history. He was born in Pergamon, in the Roman Empire's eastern provinces of Asia Minor. In the year 162 B.C., when he was thirty-three years old, he moved to Rome, where he ascended to the court as physician to the Emperor Marcus Aurelius.

In Rome, Galen wrote his first book on medical practice, the title of which revealed the message it brought. A suitable translation would be "The best physician is also a philosopher." In this book, Galen condemned the ignorant and materialistic doctors of his time and urged his colleagues to emulate Hippocrates. "Turn away from riches, decadence, and the pleasures of the leisurely life," he advised them, "and, like Hippocrates, devote yourself to the pursuit of knowledge." Although he lived in Rome, the lavish center of the Empire, and had enormous prestige there, Galen himself followed the Hippocratic example. He dedicated himself to medicine, carried out research, and wrote extensively for the benefit of other doctors. Many of his publications have survived over twenty centuries. A nineteenth-century edition of Galen's works contains twenty-two volumes. Ten thousand pages cover practically everything known in medicine at the time they were written. Hippocrates is cited more than twenty-five hundred times. The topics range from anatomy and physiology to philosophy and medical ethics, pathology, pharmacology, therapeutics, psychology, orthopedics, surgery, medical conduct, and the art of prognosis and diagnosis.

The influence of Galen on the training of doctors and the practice of medicine up to the Renaissance period, and in some subjects up to the present, was enormous. His work was based on observing nature and the critical analysis of the work of his predecessors. Foremost among these to command his respect was Hippocrates, the man he recognized as the father of medicine. Whenever one of Galen's contemporaries disagreed with his interpretations or with his therapeutic recommendations, he would react fiercely, ridiculing his adversary's position with counter-arguments inspired by Hippocrates.

Galen practiced bloodletting for the treatment of almost any ailment and he defended its use with unyielding conviction. Adopting the same rationale Hippocrates had used five hundred years earlier, he emphasized the extraordinary benefit of menstruation in relieving the periodic ills from which some women suffered. As Hippocrates had done before him, Galen based his arguments for bloodletting on the balance theory to explain the function of the human body. Galen believed that the body was formed of autonomous parts and each one of these parts had a specific function. The function of the body as a whole depended on four humors. Two of the humors, blood and yellow bile, were considered hot, while the other two, phlegm and black bile, were cold.

Blood and phlegm were damp while yellow bile and black bile were dry. Health was maintained through the equal balance of opposites and disease resulted from the dominance of one of them. The balance of the humors affected both the body and the mind. (The similar classification of the four temperaments, sanguine, choleric, phlegmatic, and melancholic, is post-Galenic.) The balance theory gave rise to the system of treatment in which opposites were the cures for reciprocal afflictions. If the patient was too hot, cooling was the proper treatment; if too dry, treat by dampening, etc. Menstruation was seen as nature's way to reestablish the harmonious humoral balance and thereby relieve the periodic ills from which some women suffered. In his arguments, Galen makes clear reference to menstruation's healing power. He quotes Hippocrates' description of a woman who was cured of severe vomiting when her menstrual flow started. Galen reasoned that if health consists in a perfect mixture (eucrasia) of the four humors in the body, and disease in a dyscrasia or unbalanced mixture, then each of the humors should, when present in excess, be capable of producing such a dyscrasia.

Galen invoked the theory of the humors, which he credited to Hippocrates, to justify therapeutic bloodletting without directly claiming that an excess of blood caused the conditions for which it was needed. Remember that Galen had no knowledge of blood circulation, although he did recognize that one part of the body communicated with another through the arteries and veins. In fact, it was fifteen hundred years after Galen, in 1682, that the English anatomist, William Harvey, first described blood circulation in his book *De Motu Cordis*. It was Harvey, marveling at the scope and depth of Galen's contributions to medical understanding, who referred to him as "the Prince of Medicine."

Despite Galen's august stature in medicine, some of his contemporaries had doubts about bloodletting and limited its use. This conservative approach followed the recommendation of the great Egyptian doctor Erasistratus, who lived in Alexandria around 300 B.C. and whose influence persisted for centuries after his death. The limitations placed on bloodletting by the followers of Erasistratus enraged Galen. In several books, he attacked their views, referring frequently to the writings credited to Hippocrates. In the first book, Galen criticized Erasistratus for recommending binding of limbs in cases of pulmonary bleeding and questions not only his competence as a doctor but also his sincerity. He ridicules Erasistratus for failing to even mention venesection for the treatment of diseases, even though at the time of his writings there had already been considerable use of the procedure, especially by Hippocrates himself.

When criticizing the followers of Erasistratus, Galen referred to them as his adversaries and lists with scorn and condescension the principal arguments against bloodletting that they use. "We have the utterances of some who say that it is difficult to estimate the amount of the evacuation, so that one is compelled either to do no good to the patient who is insufficiently evacuated, or to cause the gravest harm to the one in whom the amount is exceeded."

"For what is the difference," they say, "between unregulated phlebotomy and murder? Others maintain that an inrush of pneuma into the veins might take place from the arteries, since pneuma must follow of necessity through the [incisions] when the blood is emptied out.

"Still others say that since inflammatory conditions arise in the arteries, there is no point in emptying the veins. Even if such pronouncements might seem convincing to some, yet in relation to the truth itself they carry no conviction and are plainly false."

His attack on Erasistratus is merciless. "You must have written these things shut up in some house, never seeing a single patient; this is probably why you are ignorant of the works of nature. You are always marveling but never imitating, which makes you stupid in the last degree." Unrelenting, he continues, "Even, however, if you did not see patients yourself, you might at least have read the works of

Hippocrates and learned how many cases nature . . . brings to a crisis perfectly and faultlessly."

Galen supported his arguments by citing the views of great names in medicine who were in agreement regarding bloodletting, even if they differed on other matters. In that pre-experimentation era, these respected physicians frequently turned to nature to justify their theories: "Does she (nature) not evacuate all women every month, by pouring forth the superfluity of the blood? It is necessary, in my opinion, that the female sex, who stay indoors, neither engaging in strenuous labor nor exposing themselves to direct sunlight—both factors conducive to the development of plethora (an excess of blood)—should have a natural remedy by which it is evacuated." His attack had no limits. "If you had the intelligence to understand further what great benefits accrue to the female sex as a result of this evacuation, and what harm they suffer if they are not cleansed, I don't know how you would be able to go on wasting time and not eliminate superfluous blood by every means at your disposal."

Galen's argument on menstruation, illness, cleansing, and the virtue of blood loss is stated with no uncertainty in this blunt challenge to his adversaries. "I see myself as a town-crier shouting the truth at you, that a woman who is well cleansed is not seized with gout or arthritic or pleuritic or peripneumonic diseases, and that neither epilepsy nor apoplexy nor suspension of breathing nor loss of speech occur at any time if she is properly cleansed. Has a woman ever been known to be stricken with phrenitis, or lethargy, or a spasm, or tremor, or tetany, while her menstrual periods were coming? Or did you ever hear of a woman who suffered from melancholy or madness or headache, or from any of the major and severe diseases, if her menstrual secretions were well established? And, on the other hand, if they are suppressed, she is certain to fall into every sort of illness."

"But enough of women for the present; come now to consider the men, and learn how those who eliminate the excess through a hemorrhoid all pass their lives unaffected by diseases, while those in whom the evacuations have been restrained have fallen into the gravest illnesses. Will you not let blood from these men? Does your arrogance extend to letting so many die because you refuse to retract your mistaken notions? I would not put it past you."

"Do not suppose that your quarrel is with Hippocrates alone when he recommends the evacuation of blood, in cases where a man, through suppression of a hemorrhoid, or a woman, from suppression of the menses, falls into a rigor, or a dropsy, or any other cold disease. You are at odds too with all physicians who rely on experience. Would you not concede that the natural course anyone would take when faced with a plethora of blood was to evacuate it? Who does not know that opposites are the cure for the opposites? This is not the doctrine of Hippocrates alone; it is the common belief of all men."

Galen attacked Erasistratus and his followers not only for opposition to bloodletting but also for endorsing fasting as a medical treatment. Erasistratus wrote that: "The practice of not giving food to wounded patients during the time when inflammation is occurring is also consistent with these principles; for the veins, when emptied of nutriment, will more readily receive back the blood that has gone across to the arteries." To this, Galen replied: "In other words, fasting puts an end to inflammations. He gives no other reason for using it in inflammatory conditions than that the evacuated veins will more readily receive back the blood that has gone across to the arteries. Ye gods! Anyone who wants to empty the veins, then, must engage in a long struggle, when it is perfectly possible to achieve it without distress, and in a short time! I don't know how anyone could be caught tripping over his own feet more obviously than this."

Through the ages, medicine has not been exempt from professional disagreements, disputes, and adversarial relations, but nothing approaches the hard-hitting, *ad hominem* assault used by Galen to demolish those who were reluctant to accept his argument on menstruation, and its offshoot, therapeutic bloodletting. Considering his status in medicine, it must have been devastating to those who questioned his opinions. Galen could not have suspected that the controversy would resurface centuries later, with similar vitriolic attacks and high-spirited emotions.

Galen's Instruction Book on Venesection

At the request of colleagues who wanted a practical handbook, Galen wrote a short treatise entitled "Galen's Book on Treatment by Venesection." This provided doctors not only with technical instructions for applying bloodletting but also the theoretical basis for its use. In the introduction, Galen confirms his steadfast belief in the virtues of bloodletting and his disdain for those who cannot see its advantages in practically any ailment. The indications he advises include preventive bloodletting in the springtime, when there is a plethora of blood. In the "how-to" section, he writes that women who do not menstruate should be bled by suction of a vein in the leg. Bleeding a vein in the arm has the opposite effect, sometimes even suppressing menstruation. Frequently, bloodletting is carried out during several days to simulate a menstrual flow. In more serious cases, Galen recommends bleeding up to one pint or until the patients lose consciousness. Deaths are discounted as unfortunate accidents. For all indications, he carefully describes and justifies the venesection procedures that should be used such as which vein to cut, and how much blood to remove.

Addressing what today's physicians would call the mechanism of action, the Prince of Medicine explained that not only do the parts of the body derive their nourishment from the blood, but they are also heated by it, exactly as the warmth of a fire heats the whole house. Just as the fire in the hearth can be diminished by the indiscriminate placing of logs on it, the heat in the heart can sometimes become less or greater than normal because of the excess of blood or the lack of it. "Sometimes unnatural heat or cold develops in one particular part of the body. But these localized states of heat and cold do not extend to the whole body unless they have first affected the heart."

Believing people have more blood in springtime, Galen claimed to have cured patients who suffered chronically by removing blood at winter's end. According to Galen, only people who are temperate in their way of life could be benefited by his therapy. "Neither drunkards nor gluttons can be helped by purging or phlebotomizing. One really ought not to undertake to treat these patients, but where they are cooperative, you will help them most at the beginning of spring, first evacuating them in advance, and then leading them on to exercises and a healthy way of life."

Galen considered his opinion on the health risk of the absence of menstruation (amenorrhea) indisputable. On this subject, his point of view has prevailed over two thousand years. "Evacuation should not be deferred in these patients," states the Prince of Medicine. "It is not essential, however, to open a vein, for in fact scarifications of the ankles are sufficient to eliminate the excess, since they possess some other power to urge on the menstrual changes, just as venesection at the ankles and hams do. You should always evacuate women who suffer from suppression of the menses from the legs, either by opening a vein or by scarifying. Those of them who are of fairer complexion collect thinner blood, and hence derive the greatest benefit from scarification at the ankles. But treat those who are darker by phlebotomy, since they accumulate thicker blood. More slender and darker women appear to have larger veins, while smallness of the veins is characteristic of those who are plump and fair, and in these it is better to scarify the ankles than to cut a vein."

A crucial point which, according to Galen, was discovered and promulgated by Hippocrates, is that bloodletting only works when it is carried out on the same side as the disease or the symptom. "Those who bleed from the opposite side,"

he states, "do not help at all, and sometimes even do harm."
"A hemorrhage from the right nostril confers no benefit on
an enlarged spleen, nor does one from the left nostril benefit
the liver."

"Inflammatory conditions of the uterus are benefited
even more than those of the kidneys by the veins in the
legs being cut. There is an additional difficulty with evacuations at the elbow for they check the menstrual purges,
diverting the blood towards the upper parts of the body. By
evacuations from the legs, however, it is possible to urge on
the menses. When you wish to achieve this at the time
when the woman's period is due, start about three or four
days in advance by cutting a vein or scarifying one leg, and
draw off a little blood. On the next day evacuate in the same
way from the other leg, at the same time prescribing a reducing diet for the days on which you evacuate. But even
in women who are not on this diet," Galen advises, "mint
and pennyroyal bring on an abundant menstrual flow." He
warns, however, that sometimes the uterus bleeds from an
erosion. In these patients the aim of treatment is not the
same: "We do not wish the blood to flow as it does in the
menses; but at all costs to stanch it."

Like Hippocrates before him, the impact of Galen on
medicine was enormous and his extraordinary defense of
bloodletting for practically every ailment, based on the rationale of menstruation's relief of the burden of illness,
lasted over two thousand years, up to the twentieth century.

Bloodletting After Galen

After fifteen centuries of bloodletting as the principal therapeutic resource for all ills, at the beginning of the sixteenth
century, it became the center of a fierce controversy over
how and when it should be used. Galen's influence in medicine remained strong through the centuries. Harvey, who
discovered blood circulation about fifteen hundred years after Galen, went out of his way to avoid criticizing the

bloodletting theories of the Prince of Medicine. With his discovery, Harvey, who referred to Galen as "the Divine," could have discredited not only the practice of bloodletting but also the Hippocratic and Galenic idea of humors.

The sixteenth-century debate began with the emergence of the Arab school of doctors who did not reject Galen's idea, but practiced a modified form of bloodletting, based on conservative treatment. One aspect of the debate was the difference between revulsion and derivation. According to Galen, revulsion was evacuating the humors responsible for a localized illness, and leading them off to a healthy part of the body. In this way, Galen believed, if the illness is in the feces or in the urine, inducing emesis (vomiting) would act as a revulsion. Derivation was described as leading the humors away from their natural path to an area of the body where there was an affliction. The crucial difference between revulsion and derivation was that one approach believes in diverting the humors from the sick parts to the healthy parts, while the other diverted humors from the healthy parts to the sick ones. Obviously, this was not a simple semantic difference, easily papered over. There were other differences as well, concerning when to apply bloodletting and which side of the body to use.

The debate raged, with arguments for and against revulsion or derivation, between the right or left side of the body, between conservative and aggressive application of the treatment. The conservative Arab method predominated during the entire Middle Ages until the sixteenth century. Phlebotomy was carried out in one vein, situated as far as possible from the site of the disease, and small quantities of blood were removed. A Parisian doctor named Pierre Brissot led the opposition to this technique. He used an epidemic of pleurisy in 1514 to test the effectiveness of copious bloodletting, following the recommendations of Hippocrates and Galen. In his opinion, the results were so good that the following year he made a public announcement condemning the Arab method. This started one of the most heated medical controversies of all time, lasting almost a hundred years. It was reminiscent of Galen's assault on Erasistratus over a millennium earlier. Brissot criticized what he called the "Arab nonsense," a procedure which was so "absurd" as to remove only one or two drops from the big toe on the side opposite to the affliction. He claimed, like Galen, that in order to have an effect, a substantial amount of blood had to be drawn and it did not make any difference which side was bled.

Brissot obtained some support in Paris but the general reaction was contrary to his proposal because Parisian doctors were more inclined to use the Arab method. For some time the debate was confined to Paris, but some years later, after Brissot settled in Portugal, the controversy erupted there. An epidemic of pleurisy in the Portuguese town of Evora in 1518 gave the French doctor the opportunity to once again test the technique advised and promoted by Hippocrates and Galen. Brissot's success was so great that it incited the jealousy of the Portuguese court physician, who harshly criticized the Frenchman's proposition.

By 1525, when Brissot's rebuttal was published after his death, the medical world was divided into two factions. The Arabist followers argued that, at the onset of illness, there is little to be drawn, since the ill-fated humors had not yet accumulated in the affected region, and that the vein to be cut should be the one farthest as possible from the affected area, preferably on the opposite side of the body. Brissot's supporters insisted that in cases of lung disease, for example, the arm on the affected side was sufficiently far from the area of the illness, the chest, and that copious bleeding was beneficial. The publication of the substantial work of Brissot provoked such a violent debate in Portugal and Spain that the method advocated by him was prohibited by government mandate. The University of Salamanca, which was requested to give an opinion on the subject, favored Brissot. With support of the government, the opposition took the case to the judiciary. The Emperor, influenced by the death of a relative who had died under treatment by the Arab method, refused to support his own government.

In the midst of this hot debate, Andreas Vesalius, a Belgian doctor living in Padua, entered the discourse with the publication of a document entitled "Letter on Venesection." It was published first in Basel in 1539. A second edition was published in 1544 in Venice. The Latin text, with a translation into Dutch, was published in Amsterdam as recently as 1930 and served as a basis for further study of this interesting chapter in the history of medicine.

Vesalius' letter did not merely add theories, citations of high authorities, or personal opinions with no scientific basis. For the first time, it brought into the discussion of bloodletting facts obtained from anatomical studies of the veins dissected personally by its author. A professor at the Padua Medical School, Vesalius was to become recognized as an outstanding anatomist who earned well-deserved fame for the publication of the first great work on human anatomy. Vesalius supported Brissot and, consequently, Hippocrates and Galen. But for the first time, he challenged the infallibility of Galen with regard to anatomy.

A salutary consequence of Vesalius joining the discussion was the discovery of the valves of the heart, which enabled William Harvey to conceive of and finally describe the circulation of blood. Vesalius credited the anatomist Giambattista Canano with appreciating the important role of the valves, but not necessarily their discovery. During a visit they made together to Lake Como in 1546 to consult on the illness of Francis d'Este, patron of the still-famous Villa d'Este, Canano remarked that the heart valves prevent reflux of the blood. It was a subject quite natural to be considered when the two doctors were discussing the best way of bleeding the illustrious patient. The person who first described the structures was the Portuguese physician Amatus Lusitanus, in a criticism of Vesalius' thesis in 1551. He wrote about experimental results, which demonstrated that Vesalius' description of blood flow from the *vena cava*, the main collecting vein of the body that carries blood back to the heart and lungs, must be in error. He pointed out that as the blood reaches the heart, "there are certain portals, which open to allow the blood to flow in and close in such a way that the blood, which has gone in, can no longer return. We have determined this because it has been observed from the dissection of bodies."

The great Vesalius was obliged to respond to his critic, a Portuguese Jew. Replying in the revised edition of his anatomy textbook, he ridiculed the idea that the valves described by Lusitanus had a functional purpose in directing blood flow and attributed to them merely the function of reinforcing the walls of the veins. Vesalius' former teacher, Jacobus Sylvius, joined the debate, siding with Lusitanus and leveling stinging criticisms at his student. The famous Fallopius supported Vesalius, heaping ridicule on the Portuguese anatomist.

The debate went on through the years, contributing even further to the practice of bloodletting. The procedure retained its popularity throughout the seventeenth and eighteenth centuries and was still liberally practiced at the turn of the nineteenth century. It shortened the life of millions of its victims among whom were some of history's most notable. George Washington was bled to such a degree by his physicians that he died, probably as a result of acute anemia or from the raging streptococcus infection he had become too weakened to fight off. In retrospect, the doctors who had cared for him recognized that the bloodletting had been excessive.

This was in 1799, nearing the dawn of the nineteenth century, two thousand, two hundred years after Hippocrates legitimized and advocated the practice of bloodletting, inspired by women's menstruation.

The industrial revolution brought dramatic demographic changes. In industrialized countries both birth rates and death rates declined. As women's life expectancy increased, greater numbers reached menopause. Considering the supposed benefits that habitual bleeding brought women, the inexplicable halt of menstruation worried doctors. Many attributed whatever ailment would afflict a menopausal woman to her lack of menstruation and prescribed, with certain logic, bloodletting as a solution.

In 1857, the famous London physician Edward Tilt published a book in which he defended bloodletting as the preferred method for treating the menopause. All the symptoms of the menopause—hot flushes, headaches, dizziness, night sweats—would disappear if this imitation of nature were followed, promised Tilt.

Some doctors would use leeches to remove the excess blood from the menopausal patients. Pregnancy was another condition during which the absence of menstruation worried doctors. In order to rectify what they considered nature's failure, doctors providing prenatal care would practice bloodletting at any sign whatsoever of discomfort, including nausea, headaches, or dizziness. Incredible as it now seems, in the seventeenth century, bloodletting was the only medical means of prenatal care. One to two pints of blood was removed at each bloodletting. In some towns of Austria and Bavaria, women were routinely bled once or twice during pregnancy.

Henry Clutterbuck, a member of the Royal College of Medicine, published a book in London in 1840 entitled *On the Proper Administration of Bloodletting for the Prevention and Cure of Disease*. In it, Clutterbuck stated, "Bloodletting is not only the most powerful and most important but is also the most used of all our remedies. . . . Rarely is there a case of acute or even chronic disease in which it does not become necessary to consider the need to resort to the lancet."

In 1823, Benjamin Rush, also in London, wrote, "The common resources of the lancet, a garden, a kitchen, fresh air, cool water, and exercise, will be sufficient to cure all diseases that are present under the power of medicine." It is surely no coincidence that when the English physician Thomas Wakley founded the English-language medical journal in the same year that was to become, arguably, the world's most prestigious, he chose as its name, *The Lancet*.

Bloodletting in Modern Times

Medicine began to thrive in the United States in the nineteenth century and assumed world leadership during the twentieth century. In the second edition of the nineteenth-century book on bloodletting by Marshall Hall entitled *Research on the Morbid and Curative Effects of Loss of Blood*, the author made it perfectly clear that no other treatment was as important and as widely used as bloodletting. As medicine progressed in the second half of the nineteenth century, the excesses of bloodletting began to be recognized. However, its practice continued to be recommended even by the most renowned American physician of the turn of the century, William Osler, whose textbook on internal medicine, entitled *The Principles and Practice of Medicine*, was the main source of medical teaching at the beginning of the twentieth century. The book, first published in 1892, adopted a selective attitude, advising against bloodletting in thrombosis and cerebral embolism, but recommending the procedure in cases of manic-depressive syndrome and in various other afflictions, especially pneumonia.

America's great medical educator wrote, "In many cases, the question comes up at the outset as to the propriety of venesection. The reproach of Van Helmont that a 'bloody Moloch presides in the chairs of medicine' cannot be brought against the present generation of physicians. During the first five decades of this century, the profession bled too much, but during the last decades we have certainly bled too little. Pneumonia is one of the diseases in which a timely venesection may save life. Time and time again, in such cases have I urged free venesection, but in twelve hospital patients bled under these circumstances [a late stage of the disease] only one recovered."

That the revered Osler, within the lifetime of some centenarians living today, could recommend the use of bloodletting reveals the impotence of other approaches to curative medicine at that time and the extent to which therapeutic bleeding had been embedded in medical thought and practice. During the twentieth century, despite the long domination that the ancient belief held over medicine, the favored remedy of physicians for two thousand years was finally demystified by science and practically abolished from modern medical practice.

Bloodletting crossed the Dark Ages, the Middle Ages, the Renaissance, and the Enlightenment. Today, the procedure is only used in the treatment of hemochromatosis, a disease transmitted genetically and characterized by the accumulation of iron in the liver, pancreas, heart, and other organs, causing cirrhosis of the liver, heart failure, and impotence in men. Bloodletting is carried out weekly in patients suffering from hemochromatosis, when approximately one pint of blood is drawn, corresponding to two hundred and fifty milligrams of iron. One wonders whether physicians of later decades of the new century will react with disbelief that this form of therapy was carried into the new millennium.

For almost three thousand years of the documented history of humanity, bloodletting was an instrument of healing that, instead, shortened the lives of millions of people. Kings and queens, rich and poor, who relied on their doctors, had a high probability of dying from bloodletting. In 1925, *The Lancet* published a declaration calling the attention of doctors to the potentially fatal risks run by patients submitting to bloodletting—a technique still practiced at that time by many doctors all over the world. The teachings of Hippocrates, inspired by menstruation, reinforced by the vigorous exhortations of Galen, established bloodletting as the principal instrument of physicians for the treatment of almost all ailments from antiquity up to the twentieth century.

3

∞

Why Women Menstruate

The biological cause of the menstrual cycle is the changing cascade of hormones produced by the brain, pituitary gland, and ovary of a woman who has achieved the age of puberty, or the menarche. These chemical messengers are the product of evolutionary adaptations that have produced a system to restrict the reproductive rate to a single offspring, nurtured and protected in the woman's uterus, and nursed and cared for after birth. The result is a method of reproducing that is physiologically efficient for the individual and effective to assure continuity of the species. In more primitive vertebrates, fish or frogs for example, survival of the species is based not on nurturing, but on the production and fertilization of huge numbers of eggs, only a few of which will survive to reach sexual maturity and maintain the reproductive cycle.

How Humans Reproduce

The human female body, from the time of sexual maturation, prepares each lunar month for the possible occurrence of a pregnancy; two different sequences of events are repeated. From among the tens of thousands of immature eggs in the ovaries, several will start to develop, each within its own compartment of the ovary called the follicle. After about ten days, usually only one will continue to flourish and become fully mature, ready to be released from its follicle at about mid-cycle on the fourteenth day. As ovulation occurs, the follicle bursts with a spectacular eruption of the egg's dispersed corona of nurse cells, and the mature egg is swept from the surface of the ovary by the undulating end of the fallopian tube. Observed and photographed by scientists, this critical event in the life cycle resembles the beauty of celestial displays of distant galaxies. Fertilization can occur only if, around the time of ovulation, sperm ascend to the fallopian tube.

The arrival of the sperm triggers the completion of the process (meiosis) that reduces by half the number of the egg's chromosomes so that fusion of sperm nucleus with egg nucleus produces the normal complement of chromosomal DNA, the genetic material. There is also hereditary information provided by non-nuclear DNA found in the cytoplasm of the egg, associated with structures known as mitochondria. This component of hereditary information is totally maternal and plays a key role in programming the fertilized egg for the subsequent steps in development. Next, a slow series of cell divisions (mitosis) begins as the fertilized egg passes through the fallopian tube into the uterus. Four days after fertilization, the egg is a cluster of thirty-two or sixty-four cells, beginning to divide more rapidly. Very little development occurs while the egg remains free within the uterus. It may float unattached for one or two days and assume the form of a microscopic signet ring, with an inner mass of cells encircled by a single row of cells in alignment. This pre-embryo state is called the blastocyst. Under proper conditions, the blastocyst will nestle into the uterine wall on the fifth or sixth day after fertilization and begin to form the placenta. The inner cell mass, after several more days of mitotic divisions and internal arrangements, will become a human embryo.

Meanwhile, a second sequence is taking place to assure a safe and supportive nesting place in the uterus, if and when the blastocyst arrives. Early in the cycle of ovarian events, before ovulation, the ovary in response to hormonal signals received from the pituitary gland via the bloodstream secretes in ever-increasing amounts the female sex hormone, estrogen. This steroid molecule stimulates the lining of the uterus, the endometrium, to proliferate, and it sensitizes the cells of the endometrium, to the second ovarian hormone, progesterone. Testosterone, another steroid hormone, is also produced in small amounts and plays a role in sexual arousal. As the estrogen level reaches a peak, one of the pituitary hormones (luteinizing hormone or LH) also peaks. Specialized receptor proteins on the outer membrane of ovarian cells recognize these high hormone levels. This triggers follicle rupture and release of the mature egg at the ovary's surface. After ovulation, the ovary's vacated follicle, referred to at this stage as the yellow body or corpus luteum, begins to produce progesterone, and the production of estrogen falls off considerably before initiating a second rise later in the cycle.

The Role of Progesterone

The presence of progesterone is absolutely essential for the establishment and maintenance of a human pregnancy. Among the functions it performs are: the preparation of the uterine lining for implantation of the fertilized egg, development and maintenance of the vascular bed that becomes the maternal part of the placenta, suppression of subsequent ovulations during pregnancy, and the prevention of contractions of the uterine muscle that would dislodge a developing embryo or fetus at any stage of pregnancy. All of these are critical roles, without which human reproduction could not take place and the species could not survive. As scientists learn more about this remarkable hormone, it is no exaggeration to claim that progesterone is a hormone without which there would be no human life.

When fertilization occurs, the blastocyst signals its presence by sending an LH-like chemical message via the bloodstream to the woman's hormone system. This initiates a series of events that continues the production of progesterone by her ovaries. This is vital because without the maintenance of progesterone production, uterine contractions can start, the uterine lining sloughs off, the enlarged blood vessels rupture, and the lost blood and sloughed cells are discharged through the cervix and vaginal canal as a menstrual flow. The large protein that carries this message from the blastocyst through the maternal blood system to the woman's ovary, alerting it to continue producing progesterone, is the hormone that all pregnancy tests are designed to identify. Known technically as human chorionic gonadotropin (hCG), this pregnancy hormone can be found in a woman's blood or urine even before the first missed period, when the most sensitive tests are used.

It is the dividing fertilized egg, therefore, that controls its own destiny by producing the chemical message to avoid the oncoming menstruation in which it, too, would be lost. Averting the first menstruation is the first crisis confronting the new conceptus. Next, it must be concerned with the limited life span of the maternal corpus luteum, the production source of the essential progesterone. By the eighth or ninth week of pregnancy, when the woman's progesterone production begins to fail, the fetal placenta itself takes on this function, thus freeing itself from dependency on maternal hormones for its survival. Amazingly, at this point, if the mother's ovaries are removed, the pregnancy can continue, supported by the hormones produced by its own placenta.

What is Menstruation?

Menstrual cycles are exclusively characteristic of humans and a few other anthropoid primate species. Among all other mammalian species, a menstruation-like phenomenon occurs only in the bat and the elephant shrew. Human menstrual cycles are the result of advanced evolutionary adaptations to restrict the reproductive rate while assuring maximal chances for survival of a single newborn. All of these evolutionary adaptations have occurred in the female reproductive system. Human and non-human primate males continue to produce countless numbers of sperm throughout life, in a manner not particularly different from lower vertebrates or even invertebrates. A microscopist looking at a cross-section of a primate testis sees a structure remarkably similar to that of a frog, fish, or mouse. The primate ovary, however, is highly specialized. Perhaps the most important evolutionary adaptation is the development of the follicular structure with specialized cells that produce the essential hormones of the ovarian (and menstrual) cycle. There is also a restriction of the reproductive rate of immature germ cells to a short few months during fetal development, thus giving the anthropoid female a relatively small but carefully protected number of potential eggs, rather than the massive numbers seen in lower vertebrates. Over the course of a woman's lifetime, normally no more than five hundred eggs may be released. The remainder, well over 99 percent of the initial endowment of fifty thousand eggs at birth, gradually disintegrate within the ovary. Complete depletion of the ovary's supply of eggs by this process of atresia, signals the onset of the menopause. From these changes, the menstrual cycle has evolved and, concurrent with the development of the uterus, placentation, lactation, and maternal instinct establish the unique nature of the human reproductive system.

The human menstrual cycle, from the first day of menstrual flow to the beginning of the next flow, averages about twenty-eight days. In other primates it can range from twenty-seven to forty-two days. In all menstruating species, each month the female prepares for pregnancy by hormonal changes that cause the lining of the uterus to grow richly in vascularity and tissue thickness. Thus prepared, the uterus awaits the arrival of a fertilized egg. In a month when fertilization does not occur, the ovarian production of progesterone starts to wane a few days after ovulation and about fourteen days post-ovulation, menstruation occurs. The sloughing of the endometrium and the consequent bleeding are preceded by an increase in uterine contractility similar to that occurring during the onset of labor, or before a spontaneous abortion. The uterine contractions cause a constriction of the blood vessels, which have been developing and expanding in preparation for the formation of a placenta for the nourishing of an embryo. Closing of the blood vessels deprives the endometrium of oxygen, accelerating its structural disorganization and sloughing.

As the endometrial arterioles and capillaries rupture and the uterine cavity fills with blood, the contractions cause an emptying of the mixture of the sloughed tissue of the endometrium and the lost blood. The uterine contractions that develop during the menstrual period can attain levels of intensity as strong as contractions that develop during a miscarriage or labor. These contractions are experienced by many women and are more commonly known as cramps.

In the first post-ovulatory week of a typical menstrual cycle the uterine muscle remains quiescent under the influence of progesterone being produced by the woman's ovary. In the second week, if fertilization and early development does not take place and progesterone levels continue to fall, the uterus begins to show signs of sporadic contractile activity, similar to that observed in the last months of a normal pregnancy.

As the first day of the menstrual flow approaches, contractile activity increases both in intensity and frequency. As long as the endometrial remains and blood have not been expelled, the uterus continues to contract regularly for three to five days. The uterine muscle, or myometrium, develops an activity similar to the pattern that develops during labor when the fetus and its membranes are expelled. However, in adolescents, they tend to be painful when the cervix is slower to dilate and the expulsion of the uterine contents becomes more difficult. This causes prolonged contractions similar to muscle cramps.

The contractile activity of the uterus initiates and maintains the process of shedding of the endometrium and emptying of the uterine cavity. This activity is greatest when estrogen and progesterone reach their lowest levels. When these hormones are at their highest levels, the uterus is quiescent, allowing the egg's implantation site to become securely established. Maintenance of a high hormone level, especially progesterone, prevents uterine contractions so that pregnancy can proceed.

The uterine contents expelled during menstruation consist of a mixture of blood, endometrial remnants, and products of the tissue decomposition, as well as various secretions including cervical mucus. Menstrual blood coagulates before being expelled from the uterus. During menstruation, vasoconstriction causes immediate blood coagulation, the body's usual mechanism for stopping hemorrhage and re-establishing hemostasis. The small clots are formed principally by the transformation of a blood protein called fibrinogen into fibrin, and by the blood's platelets which aggregate under the influence of several substances including prostaglandins. By causing vasoconstriction of arteries and arterioles, and by contributing to clot formation by facilitating platelet aggregation, prostaglandins help to reduce bleeding. But there is also a negative side. Prostaglandins cause contractions of the smooth muscle tissue of the uterus. This interferes with clot formation and therefore contributes to continuing the uterine bleeding. Bleeding stops when a new endometrium develops under the stimulatory action of the rising level of estrogen, a product of the new ovarian cycle.

Normally, a woman discharges about thirty to fifty milliliters of blood during a menstrual flow, which usually lasts three to five days. There are ethnic differences. Some experts accept sixty to eighty milliliters as the outer limit of normalcy. During menstruation, a woman may lose more than one hundred milliliters of blood from the general circulation. The blood loss is no different from the bleeding that would occur if a small artery were traumatized anywhere else in the body. A menstruating woman also loses a similar quantity that is expelled by retrograde flow through the fallopian tubes into the spaces among the organs of the pelvic cavity. This blood is reabsorbed through the peritoneal and visceral walls in a process that continues for several days following the menstrual period. The presence of menstrual blood in the peritoneal cavity can be observed by ultrasonographic examinations during and after menstruation. On one hand this mechanism helps to preserve vital blood components such as iron. On the other hand, this retrograde flow can cause serious ailments such as endometriosis and infections.

Comparative Reproduction of Primates

Human beings have evolved from ancestral predecessors shared with present-day non-human anthropoid primates such as the chimpanzee and the gorilla. For a comparative evolutionist, these hominoid species can serve as models of the sexual and reproductive behavior of early man and woman. The menstrual cycles of several species of monkeys, such as the *rhesus* monkey (*Macaca mulatta*), baboons (*Papio anubis* and *Papio cynocephalus*), chimpanzees (*Pan troglodytes* and *Pan paniscus*), and gorillas (*Gorilla gorilla*), are similar to that of the human species and have the same duration of about twenty-eight days. Behavioral variations in association with ovulation and menstruation are pronounced in monkeys and baboons. At the time of ovulation, the female spends more time in proximity to males and their sexual overtures to the males become more frequent. Female chimpanzees of *P. troglodytes* develop cyclical sexual activity, accepting all adult males in the group during the ovulatory period and becoming uninterested and unreceptive for the rest of the cycle. Female chimps of *P. paniscus* are sexually receptive throughout the entire menstrual cycle, as is the human female. Although the female gorilla is receptive to males throughout her twenty-eight-day period, her sexual interest increases intensely during the two or three days of the cycle around ovulation.

In most non-human primates, the male initiates sexual

activity. Older males, who are generally stronger and more aggressive, become dominant and tend to copulate more frequently and with a greater number of females. Usually, females accept only the dominant males throughout the cycle, but during the ovulatory period, the female chimpanzee copulates with almost all adult males. Monogamy is rare among non-human primates. One exception is the gibbon (*Hylobates*) of Southeast Asia. Male and female form a constant pair after their first sexual encounter. The male guards his mate for the rest of their lives, threatening any other male who approaches her. Most gibbons live in small monogamous families composed of a mated pair and up to four dependent offspring. Among the great apes, the orangutan (*Pongo pigmaeus*) of Borneo and Java is frequently described as high in the order of non-human primates although its divergence from the human evolutionary line preceded that of the great apes of Africa. Like humans, orangutans exhibit a sexual dimorphism; males are roughly twice the size of females. Males and females live separately, each in their own territory. The only consistent social groups are comprised of females with their immature offspring. Young adult males sometimes forage with adult females for weeks or months at a time and forcibly mate with smaller, usually uncooperative females. Male–female sexual encounters vary dramatically from violent interactions between young males and adult females that can best be described as rape, to occasional long erotic treetop trysts, which usually occur between older adult males and females.

Regardless of the social structure in which they live, it is rare to find a menstruating non-human primate free-living in the wild. Ordinarily, commercial animal suppliers who provide non-human primates for medical research tend to return from a collecting trip in the wild with only adolescent animals because they are smaller, less threatening, and easier to handle. One of us (SJS) joined an expedition in northern India, seeking adult female *rhesus* monkeys. A concerted effort failed to identify among several troops of monkeys an adult menstruating female who was neither lactating nor pregnant. On the other hand, adult females kept in captivity, separated from males, menstruate regularly. Reared without contact with males, female chimpanzees have typical menstrual cycles and usually die before reaching fifty years of age, still menstruating regularly. Similar to human females, they become progressively infertile with age.

Prehistoric Woman and Menstruation

Anthropologists believe that humans and their African ape ancestors (*Pan* and *Gorilla*) diverged about five million years ago. The fossil record indicates a likely minimum date for the divergence of modern humans of 250,000–300,000 years ago. Although there is no information available regarding the patterns of sexual and reproductive behavior of early humans, they probably reproduced in the same way as non-human hominoids do today. Females separated from males would have had menstrual cycles. The males, twice as large as the females, probably copulated at will, possibly forcibly, with females and did so in the position most commonly used by present-day anthropoid primates who hold the female and penetrate from behind. However, as man evolved to an erect position as seen in *Homo erectus*, he started to copulate face to face, not, however, completely abandoning the occasional approach from behind. Perhaps the erotic interest that men associate with the buttocks of women originates in the historic past when copulation was carried out exclusively from behind. In contemporary Asian cultures, other posterior anatomical regions—the nape of the neck, behind the ears—are also associated with sexual arousal.

Similarities between primitive man and non-human primates probably extend to the practice of polygamy. In some non-human primates of today, dominant males copulate with all females while subordinate males have no sexual partners at all. In the competition to maximize genetic progeny, it is, for males, a great advantage to have priority in sexual access to females. The evolution of *Homo erectus* to *Homo sapiens* took place over two hundred thousand years ago. During this period, survival instinct driven by sexual impulse governed man's sexual behavior, as was the case for other animal species. The receptivity of the females and the sexual aggressiveness of the males determined copulation. Primatologists observe this pattern of behavior in non-human primates of today, free-living in the wild. Early human females, always in contact with males, probably became especially receptive during the days just preceding ovulation when estrogen and testosterone levels were highest. Some would have experienced the sub-fertility of puberty caused by irregular ovulatory cycles and would, therefore, copulate many times before becoming pregnant. Many would be successfully inseminated at their first ovulation. They would never experience regular menstruation but would continue to be amenorrheic (free of menstruation) during pregnancy and breast-feeding, just as they were in infancy and adolescence. The nomadic life, which demanded long and strenuous walks, may have contributed toward inhibiting ovulation in young women with few fat reserves, delaying the appearance of menstruation.

The supposition that paleolithic woman would have spent most of her life pregnant or breast-feeding is reinforced by anthropologic evidence indicating that the number of males exceeded females by the proportion of three to one. In most of the contemporary world, human females have a lower age-specific death rate than males in all age cohorts, but for early humans, the mortality of females beyond puberty must have been much higher than that of men due, principally, to reproductive causes. Estimated life expectancy in the paleolithic age was thirty-three years for men and twenty-eight for women. Women reached puberty late, generally after eighteen years of age, and died before the age of thirty. From the onset of ovulation, they were constantly pregnant, breast-feeding, or both. During pregnancy and breast-feeding they would remain anovulatory and would therefore have been free from menstruation, not only up to the menarche, but for most of the time until death, which not infrequently would have been caused by the birth of a child. Since child mortality was also high, the population did not grow to any great extent, despite these repeated pregnancies.

Some contemporary primitive cultures of Africa and Latin America maintain the reproductive behavior of their ancestors that begins as soon as sexual maturation occurs. They experience, as their predecessors did in the pre-agricultural past, alternating periods of gestation with breast-feeding on demand, remaining free of menstruation for virtually their entire life span. Anthropologists find striking differences in the patterns of reproduction among women in hunter/gatherer societies such as the !Kung San of southern Africa or the Australian Aborigines, compared to modern women in the United States. With an average of six pregnancies and nearly three years of breast-feeding per child, the hunter/gatherer woman experiences about one hundred and sixty menstrual periods in her lifetime, as compared to the average of four hundred fifty periods for a contemporary American woman. But even this reduced number of menstruations is greater than the number experienced by forager women in prehistoric times when life expectancy was shorter and the age of menarche older. Over the millennia, a progressive reduction in the age of the menarche, when menstruation begins, can be accounted for by the gradual improvement in nutrition available throughout the world, even to societies that have remained traditional and relatively isolated.

4

∞

Premenstrual Syndrome

Premenstrual syndrome (PMS) is a physical condition involving biological changes in the brain, hormone levels, and immune system prior and up to the menstrual flow starting. This syndrome has not always been understood and has only received widespread recognition in the last two decades. The alterations in both body and mind that take place in the days preceding menstruation foreshadow its arrival. We now know PMS is biological in nature, and laboratory or neurological tests can record some of these premenstrual events even if they are barely noticed or imperceptible to a woman.

Although menstruation is usually felt to be a natural and unavoidable regular occurrence, to which most women accommodate without complaint and with scarcely visible impact on their daily lives, nonetheless most women experience low-level discomfort such as bloating, fatigue, and backaches in the week before their periods. For about 30 to 40 percent of the female population, the symptoms they experience during this time can cause significant discomfort. But for 3 to 7 percent of women premenstrual syndrome means difficult bouts of emotional upheaval including fear, frustration, and rage that can have devastating effects on these women's daily lives. The most frequent PMS symptoms are fatigue (92 percent), irritability (91 percent), abdominal distention (90 percent), nervous tension (89 percent), breast tenderness (85 percent), mood changes (81 percent), depression (80 percent), and increased appetite (78 percent). By far, more women than men suffer from insomnia. A 1998 study by the U.S. National Sleep Foundation found that 71 percent of women reported that their sleep was disturbed in the premenstrual days and during the first few days of their periods. On average, women reported that menstruation disrupted their sleep two or three days each month. Before and during their periods women reported having more trouble falling asleep, waking up during the night, and feeling less refreshed when they awaken. Women blamed bloating, tender breasts, headaches, and cramps for causing them to lose sleep. In spite of the overwhelming evidence to the contrary, women's complaints about sleep deprivation and the causal factors have often been dismissed by health professionals as depression, hysteria, or emotional responses without a medical cause.

Doctors knowledgeable about the menstrual cycle, however, consider PMS an atypical depression, which differs from a true depression only because there are accompanying physical symptoms in the breasts and abdomen caused by water retention. The association with menstruation distinguishes PMS from other mental conditions that cause behavioral changes. The distinction between PMS and mental illness is important because it occurs both in women who are not mentally ill and those who are. In the latter, the symptoms of a pre-existent mental illness worsen in the pre-menstrual phase, requiring intensive measures to manage the patient during those days. While the premenstrual phase can influence the course of a pre-existing mental illness, it can also cause a dormant mental condition to become apparent during that period. Women with manic-depressive syndrome and schizophrenia experience a worsening of symptoms during the premenstrual phase. Modern scientific papers report an increase in the number of suicide attempts by psychiatric patients in this phase of the menstrual cycle.

In antiquity, the Greeks and later the Romans believed that the moon was the goddess Luna. She was associated with recurrent diseases and it was believed she would drive people insane if they offended her. Lexicographers claim that the term "lunatic" originated from the observation of the coincidence of crises in some psychiatric patients with the lunar (menstrual) cycle of twenty-eight days.

"I've had people tell me that every bad move they ever made in their lives—breaking up with perfectly good boyfriends, quitting perfectly good jobs—they made premenstrually," says Charlotte Furey, study coordinator of the University of Pennsylvania's Premenstrual Syndrome Program. The director of that program, Dr. Ellen Freeman, adds, "To argue that PMS should not be treated is analogous to saying that we should not treat depression."

Since the symptoms of PMS are associated with mood changes, some prefer to call it *premenstrual tension* (PMT). The expression *premenstrual dysphoric disorder* (PDD) has also been adopted to characterize the set of symptoms linked to behavioral changes such as depression, increased appetite (principally for carbohydrates), introspection, anxiety, and irritability. The American Psychiatric Association labeled PMS a mental disorder in 1987 and only recently have researchers begun to understand the biological causes for the behavioral symptoms.

Over the years, studies with a variety of drugs and pharmacological agents failed to reveal a definitive causal relationship. A study published early in 1998 in the *New England Journal of Medicine* was carried out by doctors at the prestigious National Institutes of Health, in Bethesda, Maryland. They concluded that women have PMS symptoms when their bodies overreact to the normal fluctuations in the levels of estrogen and progesterone during the week prior to their period. The study suggests that the brains of women with severe PMS may be genetically programmed to be more sensitive to changes in hormone levels. Women with a history of PMS experienced relief from mood problems when they were treated with a drug (LHRH analogue) that temporarily turned off their sex hormones. The PMS symptoms returned when they were given estrogen or progesterone, the principal female reproductive hormones.

Women who did not suffer from PMS showed no mood swings when undergoing the same treatment.

Premenstrual syndrome can appear in women of all ages during their reproductive years. It ends with menopause, or after ovarian failure for whatever cause, when menstruation stops permanently. For PMS sufferers, the arrival of menstrual bleeding either relieves the symptoms or can aggravate them to the point of requiring hospitalization. The idea has been passed down through the centuries since Hippocrates that the menstrual hemorrhage represents the body's natural mechanism of ridding itself of toxic substances responsible for women's periodic ailments. Following the lead of Hippocrates and reinforced by Galen, generations of physicians, including many in practice today, have assumed that premenstrual syndrome is an ailment and menstruation its cure.

Related to this is the historical belief, manifest in the taboos of different cultures and religions, that menstruation makes women unclean, requiring purification. The purification theme appears in the biblical story of David and Bathsheba. The chronicler tells us that Bathsheba "came to him, and he lay with her, just after she had purified herself from her period." Then she went home and soon after sent word to David that she was carrying his child. (It is likely there were other encounters since the chances of conception were slight at that early day in her cycle. If, for example, this had been the fifth day after her first day of bleeding, the probability of conceiving, based on current knowledge, would have been less than one chance in a hundred.) The practice of the cleansing or purifying bath, the *mikvah*, continues today in Orthodox Judaism.

The effects of PMS on mood and behavior can create problems in all aspects of a woman's life and can affect not only the woman herself, but also those around her. Some women with PMS report that they are less efficient at work, school, or in sporting competitions. They complain of depression, nervousness, insecurity, forgetfulness, and insomnia. Surveys show a correlation between PMS and marital conflicts, mistreatment of children, aggressiveness at work directed indiscriminately toward subordinates and superiors alike, excessive food intake, and alcohol abuse. Paranoia toward friends and relatives, loss of a job or promotion, separation from a husband, divorce, suicide attempts, and other acts of violence are all alleged to be consequences of the altered mental state of PMS sufferers during the premenstrual phase. In her book *The Woman in the Body*, author Emily Martin analyzes the anger a woman with PMS may express in terms of her life situation—abusive husband, exploitative job—and proposes that PMS may have a strong contextual and social component that is not addressed in the medical literature.

Studies carried out in England recorded behavioral changes in women with PMS. The survey data showed that the children of PMS sufferers became victims of their mother's inattention, aggressiveness, and lack of self-control. A mother could forget to feed her child or simply punish the child unfairly or excessively. It was observed that there was an increase in the frequency of children's visits to the pediatrician during the mother's premenstrual syndrome. The English researchers recorded a panoply of associated complaints, some minor and some very serious: inattention to cooking recipes, failed examinations, tardiness at classes or meetings, low marks at school, involvement in car accidents, mishaps at home or work, even committing crimes or felonies. The extreme cases are quite rare and should be considered in the context of society's expectations of women. They are expected to care for others, show self-control, and suppress anger so that their "misbehavior" in this regard stands out more than when men display the same errant traits. These arguments by Sophie Law in her book *Issues of Blood* are compelling.

Clearly, PMS can be an extremely serious problem for the patient and for those around her, but it should not be accepted as inevitable. Endocrine alterations and hemodynamic conditions similar to those occurring in the pre-labor phase bring about the changes associated with the syndrome. Water and salt retention cause edema in the breasts, brain, and abdomen. In addition, other substances, products of cellular metabolism that are produced during the short period of hormonal pseudo-pregnancy that precedes menstruation, are liberated into the circulation. These biochemical changes within the body are what actually cause the syndrome.

Symptomatic relief is the most frequent treatment. The edemas are treated with diuretics, by eliminating salt from the diet, other dietary restrictions or changes, the use of vitamins B6 and E, the administration of calcium and magnesium. For mood changes, tranquilizers and anti-depressive medications are prescribed. In recent years, ovulation inhibitors, such as the oral contraceptive pill, anti-estrogens, progestins, and progesterone itself have been used. The medical literature contains reports of women having resorted to the extremes of hysterectomy or even removal of the ovaries, rather than continue to endure monthly, extreme symptoms of PMS proven to be otherwise intractable.

Ovulation suppression, which prevents the development of the brief pseudo-pregnancy (with respect to hormone balance) which normally occurs in the post-ovulatory and premenstrual phase of a woman's cycle, is the most logical rationale for resolving the discomfort of PMS at its source. This approach has been attempted using either contraceptive steroids (the pill) or analogues of luteinizing hormone releasing hormone (LHRH), the small peptide hormone produced by the floor of the mid-brain that controls the release of ovary-stimulating hormones from the pituitary gland. Normally, the natural LHRH serves as a thermostat in turning on or off the reproductive hormones that result in ovulation (and influence the woman's body in many other ways). Chemically synthesized analogues of LHRH, taken by injection or nasal spray, can act as a shut-off valve, temporarily interrupting the cyclical changes in ovarian development and regression. This treatment has been shown to stop ovulation and prevent PMS symptoms in the work done at the National Institutes of Health, published in early 1998.

Katherina Dalton, a British doctor who is a specialist on premenstrual syndrome, has been publishing articles on the subject in medical literature since 1953. In her book *Once a Month*, written for the general public, she states that the cost to British industry of the problems associated with menstruation represents 3 percent of personnel costs. This national cost is low, she considers, when compared to the 5 percent in Sweden and 8 percent in the United States. In industries that employ mostly women, such as textiles and light electronics, the percentages are even higher. Texas Instruments Corporation, for example, registers a reduction in productivity of 25 percent during the premenstrual phase of their women employees. Dalton reports studies demonstrating that during the premenstrual phase there is a lessening of eye-to-hand dexterity. She refers to the testimony of a pedicurist who complained of bloating that made her hands heavy and stiff during the premenstrual phase. Professor Shoji Matsuda of Sapporo University, Hokkaido, Japan, studied the changes in a large number of biochemical and physical parameters during the human menstrual cycle. Among many other changes he observed was the loss of sensitivity in the ability to discern temperature differences by touch. Early in the cycle, when the right and left hands are placed in warm water differing by just one degree Fahrenheit, women could easily identify which hand was warmer or cooler. With the approach of menstruation the same women could not discern a difference of several degrees.

Although absenteeism associated with menstruation is related more to menstrual cramps, premenstrual symptoms may not actually stop the woman from going to her workplace, but they can diminish the quality of her work. A 1985 report claimed that the strongest indication that performance changes might be associated with the menstrual cycle comes from studies of achievement and motivation of women in competitive sports. In that study, no objective indication of performance change was otherwise seen.

However, one study on the influence of menstruation in an American factory that employed ten thousand women found that 45 percent of those seeking medical attention did so for reasons associated with the menstrual or premenstrual period. Dr. William Bickers and Dr. Maribelle Woods of the Virginia Medical School reported that 36 percent of women in the premenstrual phase used sedatives during working hours. Data from four London hospitals reveal that a disproportionate percentage of all female admissions to the emergency ward, fully one-half, occurred during the women's premenstrual phase. In every country where the subject has been studied, hospital admissions for depression and suicide attempts are more frequent during the premenstrual phase. Dr. Dalton also reports that accidents at work are another problem aggravated during the premenstrual phase.

Research carried out at the Center for Safety Studies in the United States revealed that the forty-eight hours preceding menstruation are the most dangerous because this is the time when most accidents occur. The reduction in mental alertness and difficulty in concentration explain computer glitches, typing errors, filing mistakes, and coffee spills—problems that plague many office workers. Journalists, authors, and artists report inexplicable difficulties and lack of inspiration or writer's block during this period.

In some professions, symptoms of the premenstrual phase can cause very serious problems. Dalton cites the example of an opera singer, whose vocal chords were affected by premenstrual edema that so altered the pitch of her voice that the prima donna was forced to cancel some of her concerts. Among my patients there have been many who felt professionally handicapped because of the physical or psychical changes of the premenstrual phase. A young American trapeze artist, the star of an international circus, felt so insecure, distraught, out of sorts, heavy, and slow that she was afraid she would die as the result of a mistimed leap during her dangerous presentation. She had already narrowly escaped death on several occasions, always during the premenstrual phase. As she had no stand-in to take her place, she was obliged to perform, sometimes twice a day. She sought my help to rid herself not only of the dangerous premenstrual phase but also of her menstrual period. During the days of her menstrual flow, she would feel weak, her hands would become damp and slippery, and she would be incapable of carrying out the acrobatics expected of her on the trapeze.

Another of my patients was a highly placed Brazilian judge who suffered from PMS that caused her to feel unsure of herself and emotionally unsettled. Fearful of committing an injustice, it became her nightmare to judge, condemn, and sentence defendants during the premenstrual phase. Preoccupation with this obsession brought her to my office for consultation.

For dancers and actresses in television or films, the mind and mood changes, inattentiveness, and difficulty in remembering lines and gestures can make performing or filming on those days impossible. Some of the most successful actresses have insisted on having clauses in their contracts releasing them from work during the premenstrual phase or during menstruation. The loss or a reduction in the senses of taste or smell can be a problem for chefs. Stories are legendary about bakers who are surprised when the cake sinks or burns because of their premenstrual distraction or forgetfulness. The disastrous journey of the Russian astronaut Valentina Tereshkova ended abruptly in 1973 when she had to be brought back to Earth after only three days because she began to menstruate excessively and there was no apparent way to control or stop the flow.

About 65 percent of patients with PMS develop both

emotional and physical symptoms. Only 5 percent report physical symptoms alone, without an emotional component, and around 40 percent suffer from mental symptoms with no physical component. The most important physical symptoms are those related to salt and water retention. This is responsible for abdominal bloating, breast tenderness with or without a perceptible increase in breast volume, pain in the hips, edema in the hands or feet, and weight increase. Water retention is obvious in many cases but in some patients it is not apparent. In these cases the symptoms are caused by the displacement and accumulation in tissues of fluids from the blood or from cells throughout the body.

A greater intake of salt-containing foods and carbohydrates contributes toward the increase in weight and edema because the increase in the intake of solids is generally accompanied by an intake of liquid. However, even when dietary restrictions are followed, many PMS victims still complain of breast tenderness, abdominal distention, and hip or back pain. To prevent premenstrual edema, doctors usually prescribe dietary restrictions including lower salt use and the use of diuretics. Some recommend greater water intake in the days before the symptoms are expected to appear. Anti-inflammatory medication, especially aspirin, is frequently used and can relieve physical symptoms such as breast pain.

Headaches, pain in the joints, back, breasts, and abdomen are the physical symptoms experienced most frequently by women who suffer from PMS, but pain can also occur in the legs, the neck, or in the whole body, as if the victim had suffered a beating. Non-steroidal anti-inflammatory drugs (NSAIDs) such as ibuprofen are frequently prescribed for the pain because they inhibit the synthesis of prostaglandins, the bodily substances most directly involved in causing the kind of pain that occurs during the premenstrual phase.

The pain associated with migraine generally receives a different kind of treatment because it originates through a different mechanism. Migraine is a severe headache, generally accompanied by nausea, gastrointestinal problems, and extreme sensitivity to light (photophobia) and noise (phonophobia). The headache can be preceded by visual disturbances called scotomas. Various factors can provoke a migraine attack: chocolate, cheese, red wine, physical and emotional stress, and sleep deprivation are among the most frequent reported by patients. In premenstrual migraine, none of these factors need be present but they can precipitate or aggravate the condition. The treatment is carried out with analgesics, ergot derivatives, caffeine and, more recently, sumitriptane, the first of a new class of agents which work through interfering with one of the body's neural transmitter substances (serotonin) involved in transmitting information from nerves to the brain. This class of drugs is proving to be extremely efficient for temporary relief of premenstrual migraine headaches. Initially introduced for use as an injection, it is now available in long-acting oral tablets or by nasal spray.

Sleep disorders associated with menstruation are due to biological phenomena and hormone balance disruption, and should not be overlooked or ignored. Sleep experts recommend habit-forming sleeping pills for only severe sleep disorders. Endocrine therapy can help by preventing the wide fluctuations in estrogen and progesterone levels that are probably the biological basis for premenstrual sleep deprivation. Menstruating women who suffer from sleep disorders should be encouraged to schedule extra time to catch up on sleep.

Emotional and mood changes are treated with light tranquilizers, anti-depressive medication, as well as with the so-called mood stabilizers such as lithium carbonate and some anti-convulsants. For patients with mental illness, both those who only suffer symptoms during the premenstrual phase and others who have an underlying mental illness whose symptoms worsen during the premenstrual phase, the treatment is carried out with anti-psychotic drugs or neuroleptic medication. Other forms of treatment for behavior and mood changes include an endocrine approach and psychotherapy. The use of hormones, initially proposed by the aforementioned Katherina Dalton, consists of the administration of progesterone suppositories, injections, or pills, and is based on the assumption that the syndrome is provoked by a deficiency of that hormone, a hypothesis that has not been confirmed by scientific data.

An alternative is treatment with estrogen, an apparent paradox if, in fact, an excess of estrogen causes the syndrome, as early specialists in the treatment of PMS, including Dr. Dalton, proposed. Nevertheless, this endocrine approach can provide relief of symptoms. The reasoning behind estrogen treatment is the possible inhibition of ovulation that can be achieved either with pure estrogen or with estrogen combined with progesterone. Ovulation can also be inhibited for several months by injections of long-acting progestins, such as medroxyprogesterone acetate, at adequate doses. Recently, we have been successful in the development of under-the-skin capsules that can inhibit ovulation for a year or longer, an approach that may prove to be extremely valuable for some PMS sufferers, provided that they are not planning to become pregnant until after discontinuing this mode of treatment.

Psychotherapy has been used when the various treatments proposed do not resolve the problem or when the patient does not accept them, preferring psychiatric consultation. Despite all these forms of treatment, relief of symptoms is sometimes not achieved. In such cases, with women desperate for relief from the monthly symptoms they experience with PMS, ovarian ablation by the use of medication, radiation, or even surgical ovariectomy has been the approach of last resort.

Mental changes can lead sufferers of PMS to cause harm to themselves or others. Obviously, the hormonal changes that lead to extreme abnormal behavior in a woman with severe PMS are beyond her control. This reasoning has led some women to use the uncontrolled symptoms of PMS as a defense in criminal proceedings. In an article published in the *The Lancet*, Katherina Dalton related the story of three women who alleged diminished responsibility as one of the attenuating factors in cases of murder, arson, or armed robbery. In all three cases, the criminal behavior occurred during the premenstrual phase. Each woman had no previous criminal record and lived compatibly with their families. Following Dr. Dalton's recommendation, in each case the magistrate agreed to have the three women receive progesterone therapy. Subsequently, none of them repeated their atypical criminal behavior.

Dr. Dalton served as an expert witness in three other cases in London. In the most famous of these cases, *Regina* v. *Smith*, the defense managed to have the accusation against Mrs. Smith changed from premeditated murder to manslaughter. Mrs. Smith, a cocktail waitress, had previously been sentenced thirty times for crimes ranging from theft to invasion of property, arson, and armed robbery. Despite this criminal history, or perhaps because of the erratic, aggressive, and apparently irrational mode of behavior, the judge accepted the defense attorney's argument that his client became an aggressive and irrational person every month during her premenstrual phase. He allowed Mrs. Smith to avoid imprisonment, conditional on accepting progesterone injection therapy. Some time later, Mrs. Smith was again brought to trial for threatening and assaulting a police officer. When the assault occurred it was alleged that the accused had not been taking progesterone as prescribed. This time, the defense argument that Mrs. Smith acted aggressively during the premenstrual phase because of PMS was not successful in having the charges reduced, but the judge did reduce her sentence. She was allowed to remain free again under the condition that she resume adequate treatment. In fact, in this case Dr. Dalton's progesterone treatment apparently did not cure or even diminish her patient's symptoms. It may have made them worse. An American gynecologist who treats women with severe cases of

PMS believes that treatment with progesterone or progestins can destabilize psychological equilibrium and must be undertaken only by a rigorously watchful physician.

Another case occurred in the English town of Norwich. A woman was accused of killing her lover by deliberately running him over with her car. She was convicted, but received the lenient sentence of twelve months under supervised detention, because her doctor testified that the patient was suffering from a serious form of PMS. Dr. Dalton also testified for the defense in the Norwich case. Her role as an expert witness in these cases, incidentally, indicates the esteem in which she is held as an authority on PMS. In Britain, unlike the United States, it is the magistrate, using objective advice from medical authorities, and not the plaintiff or defense team of lawyers, who decides who is qualified to give expert witness on medical issues.

Attempts at using PMS as a defense or as an attenuating circumstance are, however, not always successful. In the United States, the feminist movement took a decisive stance against this defense strategy. Feminists were concerned that acknowledging menstruation-related behavioral changes—especially the existence of irrational moments in women's behavior—could be harmful to women in many legal, professional, and social situations.

What is harmful to women is PMS itself, which as well as causing discomfort, pain, depression, and other mental anguish, can also create one more cause for discrimination against women in the workplace. Women with PMS should be entitled to paid leave on days when they feel their symptoms are incompatible with proper job performance. Moreover, women involved in legal proceedings should not be deprived of this defense, since it is a fact that the symptoms of PMS, including mood and mental changes, are beyond their control.

5

∽

Menstrual Cycle–Related Disorders

Several disruptive diseases or conditions can occur during menstruation for many women. These are known as catamenial diseases to indicate their monthly recurrence. They are caused by immunological, hemodynamic, hormonal, and metabolic changes that occur during menstruation. Preexisting chronic illnesses can flare up; some during the premenstrual phase, others during menstruation itself. The most common of these menstrual cycle–related disorders is dysmenorrhea, or menstrual cramps. For many women, this can be an incapacitating affliction. For others, while tolerable, it is a monthly problem they dread. Migraine is the next most frequent catamenial condition and this complex syndrome can also be life-limiting. Endometriosis, a serious chronic disease, is actually caused by menstruation. Uterine lining cells sloughed off at the time of a woman's period are discharged through the fallopian tubes into the pelvic cavity where they attach themselves to pelvic organs. Each month, these endometrial implants grow in response to hormonal changes of the cycle. Endometriosis affects about one in ten women and can be extremely painful. Frequently, it is the reason for pelvic pain and painful sexual intercourse (dyspareunia) and is a major cause of difficult to treat infertility. Additional conditions that can take on a catamenial character include asthma, insomnia, arthritis, epilepsy, and others that are exacerbated by menstruation. This chapter will discuss these disorders and their relation to a woman's menstrual cycle.

Dysmenorrhea

The most common disorder associated with menstruation is dysmenorrhea (cramping), or painful menstruation. The cramping, which for some women can be so intense as to require hospitalization, is usually the result of irregular and prolonged uterine contractions caused by estrogen hyperstimulation. These contractions result in a reduction of oxygen in the uterine muscle (myometrium) and, consequently, intense spasmodic pain (cramps). Nausea, diarrhea, sweating, dizziness, and fainting can accompany severe dysmenorrhea. The condition can become quite disruptive and can prevent a woman from carrying out her usual daily activities.

Dysmenorrhea is more common in young women, particularly adolescents, whose anovulatory menstrual cycles are associated with high levels of estrogen production by the ovary. Although beginning at puberty or soon thereafter, the condition can plague a woman throughout her life. Very few women have the good fortune to never experience menstrual cramps during the reproductive years. Congenital malformations of the uterus, tumors in the reproductive organs, endometriosis, or adhesions as a result of pelvic inflammatory disease or previous surgery can all contribute to dysmenorrhea. Menstrual cramps, under these circumstances, can be considered but one symptom associated with an underlying cause that should be diagnosed and treated. When the cause is endometriosis, pelvic pain is usually the primary and principal symptom. Most often, however, no underlying pathological condition or anatomical anomaly is present or can be discerned. Dysmenorrhea can be classified as either spasmodic or congestive. Spasmodic cramps, which affect mainly younger women, appear on the first day of bleeding, come in waves and disappear, only to return soon again with equal intensity. Congestive dysmenorrhea is characterized by intense pain before bleeding begins. It is usually seen in older women.

There are naturally occurring substances that influence the smooth muscle of the uterus to contract, when needed. Oxytocin, for example, a hormone produced in the pituitary gland, is involved in the initiation of labor at the end of a pregnancy. Prostaglandins are involved in several physiological processes of the reproductive system. As progesterone levels rise late in a woman's cycle, prostaglandin levels increase and play a key role in the initiation of menstrual contractions. Scientific studies have demonstrated that women who suffer from dysmenorrhea have elevated levels of at least one type of prostaglandin in their menstrual blood. Elevated levels can also be found in their endometrial tissue.

Most women can obtain relief with the use of aspirin or other inhibitors of prostaglandin synthesis, such as ibuprofen and similar non-steroidal anti-inflammatory drugs (NSAIDs). The new class of pain-control drugs referred to as COX-2 inhibitors should be an excellent addition to the array of possible treatments. These compounds also relieve pain by inhibiting prostaglandin synthesis, but appear to avoid the gastrointestinal symptoms that can accompany the frequent use of NSAIDs. Some women require stronger medication.

The oral contraceptive pill can be used to control severe dysmenorrhea by eliminating menstruation. The uterine bleeding associated with the cyclical use of oral contraceptive pills differs from a woman's regular menstrual bleeding. It has aptly been referred to as a pseudo-menstruation because it is actually a simulation of the real physiological event, brought about by totally different circumstances. Instead of ordinary menstruation, women using the pill experience withdrawal bleeding due to an abrupt drop in the level of external hormones reaching the uterus (hormone deprivation). This can result in a reduction in the pain of dysmenorrhea or even total disappearance of cramps. For women suffering from spasmodic dysmenorrhea, drugs of the type used to halt contractions during premature labor can be effective.

Migraine

Migraine ranks just behind dysmenorrhea in frequency of symptoms associated with menstruation. It is more common in women than in men and is usually seen in women during their reproductive years. There is ample reason to conclude that migraine attacks are associated with changes in reproductive hormone status. Women report that migraines occur primarily around the time of menstruation. The frequency of episodes decreases during pregnancy, and the condition tends to improve by the time a woman reaches menopause.

The migraine pattern of symptoms usually occurs prior to the actual start of the menstrual flow and is considered part of premenstrual syndrome in those who experience it. In some adolescent girls, migraine symptoms with no other symptoms of PMS can occur with the first menstrual period. The migraine experience often begins with photophobia (aversion to light) and visual disturbances such as spots and light flashes that dance around the visual field in various directions. This phase is followed by visual impairment, called scotoma. One part of the visual field darkens, and the sufferer is able to see only a part of what she is looking at. Occasionally, vision may be totally compromised, causing transient blindness. These visual disturbances are often followed by gastrointestinal symptoms, such as nausea or vomiting, and finally the intense migraine headache, which can last for several days. Ergot derivatives, caffeine, and more recently, agents that directly modulate the transmission of neural impulses in the brain (serotonin agonists), can be effective in the treatment of migraine symptoms.

Asthma

Nearly one-third of asthmatic women develop bronchial spasms during menstruation. In the majority of sufferers, the crisis begins in the premenstrual phase and can last through the entire menstrual period. The association of asthma with the menstrual cycle has probably been observed since antiquity, but it was only in this century that well-documented reports on the relationship began to appear in the medical literature; the first was in 1938. Women who develop crises of asthma during the premenstrual phase suffer from a more severe form of the illness than those who, although asthmatic, do not experience bronchial spasms either in the menstrual or premenstrual phase. Bronchial spasms occur more frequently in ovulatory cycles than in cycles when no ovulation occurs. This is an important clue as to the importance of hormone levels at the time of the spasm.

A study done in Sweden revealed that both about one-quarter of asthmatic women who developed crises during the premenstrual phase of the cycle and almost three-quarters of women who developed asthma during menstruation itself had a past history of hospitalization due to asthma. This suggests a more serious asthma affliction when it is associated with menstruation. An asthma attack during menstruation may be the result of the sudden reduction in the levels of steroid hormones, estrogen and progesterone. Normally, these hormones together exert an immunosuppressive effect during pregnancy, essential to prevent the rejection of the genetically unique embryo or fetus. When menstruation occurs, an indication that pregnancy has not been established, the drop in hormone levels prompts the release of the immune system from its suppression. This causes a cascade of bodily changes affecting levels of histamine, nitric oxide, specialized cells known as mast cells, prostaglandins, and other components of the body's normal milieu. One or more of these changes could be the trigger for an asthma attack.

Menstrual Thrombocytopenia

Thrombocytopenia is a disease characterized by a dangerous reduction in the number of platelets, a blood component that plays a vital role in blood clotting. When platelet levels in the blood fall to very low levels, there is a constant risk of hemorrhage. Although various types of thrombocytopenia have long been recognized in medicine, catamenial thrombocytopenia was first described as recently as 1989. The platelet count falls only during a woman's period, and causes a longer and heavier than usual menstrual flow. The platelet level returns to normal in mid-cycle, around the fourteenth day. Women with a deficiency of other important factors for blood coagulation risk dangerously excessive bleeding during menstruation since, after the flow begins, it does not always cease spontaneously and can last for many days, or even weeks. This condition, menorrhagia, can be life-threatening if left untreated. It can be caused by reasons other than low platelet counts. Women with large uterine myomas (benign fibroids in the uterine wall) or those with hypothyroidism are particularly likely to suffer from menorrhagia. In fact, a history of long and profuse menstrual bleeding, although usually the result of fibroids, is a signal to physicians to check a woman's thyroid status.

Porphyria

Porphyrias are a group of hereditary disorders caused by enzymatic defects in the biochemical process leading to the formation of hemoglobin, the oxygen-carrying component of red blood cells. Manifestation of the disease is caused by the accumulation in the tissue of toxic products that form as a result of the enzymatic deficiency. Symptoms vary according to the tissue or organs most affected and include neuro-psychiatric manifestations, abdominal pain, neuropathies, and photo-dermatitis (skin sensitivity to light).

The steroid hormones of the ovary are considered causal agents of attacks, particularly in the case of acute intermittent porphyria. This condition, aggravated during menstruation, is caused by a genetic defect that results in the blocking of an enzyme involved in the formation of the heme portion of the hemoglobin molecule. Whenever there is an increase in hemoglobin production, the defect results in a build-up of heme precursors, resulting in an acute attack of porphyria. Premenstrual attacks of porphyria may be suppressed by the use of analogues of the brain hormone LHRH, which inhibits gonadotropin release and therefore reduces or prevents secretion of sex hormones.

Arthritis

Flare-ups of rheumatoid arthritis in women may fluctuate rhythmically at intervals of approximately twenty-eight to thirty days, coinciding with the duration of the menstrual cycle. The symptoms of arthritis worsen in the premenstrual phase, remain aggravated during the menstrual period, and diminish without requiring medication at about mid-cycle, when hormone changes bring about ovulation. The symptoms frequently worsen again during the ensuing premenstrual phase. When a pregnancy is established, the symptoms can completely disappear. The use of steroid hormones, such as oral contraceptive pills, that mimic some of the endocrine changes of pregnancy can cause a reduction or even complete disappearance of the joint pain and swelling characteristic of arthritis.

Epilepsy

The correlation between epilepsy and menstruation has been known for more than a century and has been recorded frequently by neurologists who specialize in treating this disease. An extensive study on this subject was published by Dr. J. Laidlaw in *The Lancet* over forty years ago. His article reported observations of nearly a thousand epileptic women during almost ten thousand menstrual cycles. Menstruation-related seizures occurred in 72 percent of patients. A more recent comprehensive review of catamenial epilepsy was published in 1980. It reported that at least 50 percent of women with epilepsy experienced their first convulsive seizure with the onset of their first menstrual period. Electroencephalograms (EEGs) taken in the premenstrual phase confirm this correlation. In a subset of the patients studied, EEG abnormalities were more abundant in the pre-ovulatory phase when estrogen levels were higher. Another 1980 publication reported on four years of observations of sixty-nine women with a diagnosis of epilepsy. Fifty-eight percent of the women experienced convulsive seizures premenstrually and 9 percent continued to have seizure activity during menstruation.

Hormones of the reproductive system influence seizure disorders. For a woman with epilepsy, this influence often manifests itself at the time of menarche. Many women with epilepsy have seizure activity only at the time of menses, in concert with progesterone withdrawal. Another frequently observed pattern involves a clustering of seizures around ovulation, in association with peak estrogen levels. Hormone fluctuations of menopause can also trigger changes in seizure activity. Due to the pro-convulsant property of estrogen, women with epilepsy may experience a worsening of seizures when estrogens are prescribed for birth control or as post-menopausal hormone replacement therapy.

The usual anti-epileptic drugs can influence the rate of metabolism of estrogens. These drugs increase the breakdown of contraceptive hormones in the body and can, therefore, reduce the effectiveness of birth control pills. They do this because they affect a liver enzyme system, known as the cytochrome P450 system, which is involved in the metabolism of estrogen. This problem can be addressed easily by increasing the estrogen dosage in the pill to compensate for the more rapid clearance. Unfortunately, most providers who prescribe oral contraceptives for women with epilepsy do not follow this guideline. A 1996 survey of neurologists and obstetricians who treat epileptic women of child-bearing age revealed that only 4 percent of the neurologists and 21 percent of the obstetricians knew of the interaction between the most common anti-epileptic drugs and oral contraceptives.

Anti-epilepsy drugs that influence the hepatic cytochrome P450 enzymes include phenobarbital, carbamazepine (Tegretol®), phenytoin (Dilantin®), primidone (Mysoline®), and topiramate (Topamax®). These drugs can also interfere with contraceptives that are based on progestins only, such as medroxyprogesterone acetate (DepoProvera®) and levonorgestrel pills, implants (Norplant®), or intrauterine systems (Mirena®). Newer anti-epilepsy drugs, gabapentin (Neurontin®), lamotrigine (Lamictal®), and tiagabine (Gabitril®) have no effect on this enzyme system and do not interfere with hormonal contraceptive effectiveness.

Women with true catamenial epilepsy are first treated with conventional anti-epilepsy drugs for controlling menstruation-related seizures. However, some physicians have reported improved catamenial seizure control with the use of DepoProvera®, which inhibits ovulation and menstruation, and which simultaneously may reduce the changes in the brain that lead to epileptic activity. If these patients are also receiving cytochrome P450–inducing anti-epileptic drugs, they may need to receive DepoProvera® injections more frequently to maintain the desired suppression of ovulation and menstruation.

Insomnia and Hypersomnia

Both insomnia and narcolepsy-like drowsiness occur in some women during the premenstrual phase. Difficulty in sleeping is the more common experience. Sleep deprivation can be so extensive as to become debilitating. A syndrome of hypersomnia which only responds to treatment with continuous use of hormonal contraceptives (for the suppression of menstruation) was reported in 1975 and confirmed by Swedish doctors in 1982. The percentage of rapid eye movement (REM) sleep associated with dreaming has been reported to be higher in the pre-ovulatory phase of the cycle. During the premenstrual phase and menstruation, dreams tend to be more unpleasant. There is evidence that a psychiatrist can determine the cycle phase based on the dream content of psychoanalytic patients.

Menstrually-Related Pneumothorax

The first case of spontaneous pneumothorax (leakage of air into the lung cavity) associated with menstruation was reported in medical literature in 1958. This is an extremely rare event and over the subsequent forty years, only seventy cases of this condition, which can cause partial lung collapse, have been documented. Depending on the degree of escaping air, the condition can cause simply a cough with slight discomfort or an intense difficulty in breathing along with chest pain. It can cause fainting and has even been reported to be fatal.

In more than 90 percent of women affected, spontaneous menstruation-related pneumothorax occurs on the right side. It happens only during menstruation and disappears at the end of the period. These characteristics contrast with pneumothorax that is not menstrually-related, which can occur in women independent of menstruation. This type of spontaneous pneumothrorax is up to ten times more frequent in men than in women and usually affects the left side of the thoracic cavity. When it occurs in association with menstruation, the afflicted women are usually in their thirties. Non-menstrually-related pneumothorax occurs more frequently in adolescence and in menopause.

When menstrually-related pneumothorax occurs, there are various theories to account for the intermittent presence of air in the thoracic cavity. One is that air enters through the genital tract, then penetrates the thoracic cavity through defects in the diaphragm. In support of this theory are cases of women who had episodes associated with menstruation and also developed pneumothorax during sexual intercourse.

After tubal ligation, neither type of episode recurred. On the other hand, in one study only five patients out of forty-three with menstrually-related pneumothorax had any macroscopic evidence of a diaphragmatic defect. A more recent theory proposes that a causal factor for pneumothorax is an increase in blood levels of prostaglandins during menstruation. Since some prostaglandins can trigger bronchial spasms, air could escape from lung cells that rupture during the spasm, causing pneumothorax. There is little evidence in support of either postulate. The most widely accepted theory suggests that the cause is the presence of pulmonary endometriosis. Orifices or fistulas of endometriotic implants could also form on the diaphragm of patients with endometriosis.

Myomas

Myomas or fibromas are benign uterine tumors which occur in approximately 40 percent of reproductive-age women. Although they are not caused by menstruation, it is during the menstrual period that myomas cause most discomfort to women. They are of concern because they can cause an increase in menstrual flow and can prolong the duration of menstruation. The hemorrhages (menorrhagea) that occur in some patients with myomas frequently demand surgical intervention, either for the removal of the fibroid tumor or of the uterus itself. Patients who do not undergo surgery run a serious risk of developing anemia. The alternative for these women is to suppress menstruation for months or even for years.

Menstruation and Chronic Disorders

During menstruation, women can experience an aggravation of chronic disorders such as thyroid disease, problems of blood coagulation, and other metabolic abnormalities. Skeleto-muscular and joint complaints can get worse. The control of diabetes is more difficult around menstruation. Consequently, diabetic coma occurs more frequently at this time. Chronic infectious diseases, such as herpes or human papilloma virus, can flare up when the body's immunological defense is weakened. Scarlet fever, pancreatitis, hepatitis, influenza, pneumonia, and typhoid fever have all been reported occuring more frequently in the premenstrual phase. Even appendicitis appears to be more frequent during this time. Twice as many non-elective surgical procedures on women are carried out during the seven to ten days of the premenstrual and menstrual phases combined than during the rest of the menstrual cycle.

Anemia

In terms of absolute numbers of individuals, anemia is undoubtedly the disease most often affected by menstruation. Women with anemia have a significant reduction in red blood cells and a corresponding decrease in the oxygen-carrying capacity of the blood. For countless malnourished women around the world already suffering from chronic anemia, the blood loss associated with normal menstruation causes depletion in iron stores that can worsen the condition. For these women, anemia must be recognized as a potentially serious consequence of repetitive menstruation.

Other women can also be at risk. When menstruation volume is excessive, for example because of uterine fibroids, blood loss can be serious even for otherwise healthy, well-nourished individuals. With proper diagnosis and adequate medical or surgical care, these women can be treated successfully and red cell indices restored to normal. This type of care is not always available, however, particularly in the world's economically deprived regions. Consequently, excessive uterine bleeding can rapidly lead to severe anemia.

Once referred to as chlorosis characterized by pallor and lethargy, and romanticized in literature as a forlorn state in young women resulting from unhappy love affairs, anemia can be a life-threatening matter. It is caused by a reduction in the number of red blood cells resulting in a deficiency in the quantity of hemoglobin. Since hemoglobin is the principal carrier of oxygen to tissues, an anemic person suffers from a deficiency of oxygenation (hypoxia) at the cellular level. This reduces the efficiency of practically all the organs, particularly the brain and muscles, causing somnolence, loss of memory, learning difficulty, fatigue, and weakness.

Although many forms of anemia exist, the greatest number of people with anemia suffer from iron deficiency caused either by lack of iron in the diet or chronic blood loss due to parasitic infection or other causes of internal bleeding, typically from the gastrointestinal tract or the uterus. The dietary inadequacy results in insufficient replacement of iron stores. The hematological manifestations of chronic blood loss are those of iron-deficiency anemia.

Other types of anemia are hereditary. Sickle-cell anemia, for example, affecting African populations primarily, is a genetic defect that causes low oxygen-carrying capacity and abnormal destruction of red blood cells. Thalassemia is a disease that is concentrated among Mediterranean populations, but is also widely found in Asia. The principal disability in this genetic disease is failure to produce red blood cells with normal hemoglobin content. Women with the genetic constitution for a mild version of the condition survive to adulthood. They would be expected to suffer further from the periodic blood loss of menstruation but, paradoxically, they demonstrate the ability to increase iron absorption and retain larger iron stores than normal women. This gives them protection against iron-deficiency anemia.

It is estimated that approximately 30 percent of the world's six billion people are anemic. About half of those suffering from anemia, around one billion individuals, have iron-deficiency anemia. In some less-developed regions of Africa, Asia, and Latin America, most of the population suffers from anemia. Even in the more advanced, economically privileged countries of the world, 20 percent of women who menstruate regularly are anemic. Although diets deficient in iron can result in anemia, the condition is rarely caused by a dietary deficiency alone because the body is very efficient in conserving iron. In fact, no physiological pathway for the removal of iron exists. Very little iron is required to replace the loss that occurs through the shedding of body cells or through menstruation. Under normal conditions, 90 percent of the iron required to replace loss comes from the recycling of iron from aging blood cells whose hemoglobin decomposes, thus returning iron to the body's stores via the transfer protein, transferrin. Because of menstruation, the loss of iron by women is about double that of men. Normally, these losses are closely balanced by daily absorption of about 10 percent of ingested iron. An increase in the demand for iron due to growth spurts, pregnancy, or hemorrhage can boost iron absorption to about 20 percent. Frank iron deficiency can increase absorption to between 30 and 40 percent of the amount ingested. Absorption decreases, as required.

In infancy, the quantity of iron in the body is the same for both sexes. At puberty, these values start to drift apart, and men carry a larger iron load than women. This difference is reflected when measured in terms of hemoglobin per milliliter of blood. Ferritin and transferrin, the blood proteins that act as carriers of iron, also increase to higher levels in males than in females. At thirty years of age, women maintain a level of ferritin of around twenty-four micrograms per milliliter of blood while in men levels increase to ninety-seven micrograms. The ferritin level of men of age sixty rises to nearly one hundred thirty micrograms, more than 50 percent higher than that of women that age.

The marked and significant differences between men and women, particularly during the reproductive years, are explained by gene action, menstruation, and by the anabolic action of the male hormone. It has been estimated that the blood loss caused by menstruation creates an increased necessity for women of about one milligram of iron daily and around five milligrams of ferritin per day. Blood loss during menstruation has been measured in different countries with variable results that range from twenty-four milliliters in Egypt to fifty-seven milliliters in Japan. The mean value of blood loss found in studies carried out by the World Health Organization in various countries was around thirty-two milliliters (about one fluid ounce). These studies exclude the values for women using various birth control methods, such as oral contraceptives. The periodic bleeding of pill users is a pseudo-menstruation due to the pill-taking schedule— three weeks on, one week off. The bleeding experienced by women on the pill is considerably less than that of a regular menstrual flow; in some cases it is only barely perceptible. Women who use the intrauterine device (IUD) are also not included in the WHO average of thirty-two milliliters of menstrual blood flow. On the average, IUD users tend to bleed more than an average menstruation, sometimes losing more than eighty milliliters. The older and larger IUDs, such as the Lippes Loop, are associated with heavier bleeding while with the modern, copper-bearing IUDs cause less blood loss. Very little bleeding occurs when a woman uses a progestin-releasing intrauterine system, such as Mirena.

Iron deficiency occurs when the rate of loss or utilization of iron exceeds its rate of assimilation. Infants should receive iron supplementation because breast milk is a marginally adequate source of iron, and cow's milk has an even lower iron content. The increased demand for iron during adolescence is often accompanied by poor dietary habits resulting in the consumption of foods with low iron content. At a time when they most need iron, adolescents tend to prefer sweets or greasy fast foods while avoiding iron-rich vegetables. Among the elderly and the poor, financial constraints often produce a similar pattern of inadequate iron intake. Diets that consist predominantly of grains or cereals do not provide adequate quantities of iron. Populations that eat cooked wheat almost exclusively, such as some regions of Northern Africa, experience growth retardation and a delay in sexual maturation. The added burden of blood loss due to parasites such as hookworm makes iron deficiency a problem of staggering proportions. In each of these circumstances, the deficiency can be prevented by nutritional supplementation with iron and zinc.

Pregnancy and growth spurts are associated with relatively high blood plasma volume. This hemodilution results in low hemoglobin levels and low blood viscosity. Despite this state of physiological anemia, reduction in the quantity of hemoglobin in the circulation does not take place. What actually happens is a corresponding increase in the quantity of iron or in the number of red blood cells containing hemoglobin. Therefore, the apparent anemic state disappears in these circumstances when the blood volume returns to normal.

Estrogenic hormones and oral contraceptives increase the concentration of ferritin, the protein that stores iron in the body and the related protein, transferrin, that carries iron to the red blood cells and other tissues. Thus, estrogens play an important role in the mobilization of iron reserves that occurs during pregnancy and during adolescence when women begin to menstruate.

Protecting women against iron deficiency and anemia is vital. Although individuals with mild anemia are often asymptomatic or simply show the characteristic pallor of the condition, iron levels do not have to be extremely low to affect the brain, causing indifference, somnolence, memory loss, and learning difficulties. Dr. Ann Bruner and other pediatricians at the Johns Hopkins Children's Center tested the blood of more than seven hundred girls attending schools in Baltimore and discovered that nearly a hundred had levels of iron below normal but not so low as to be considered clinically significant. Dr. Bruner treated half these girls with iron as if they were anemic (two hundred sixty milligrams of iron daily for eight weeks or seventeen times the amount present in ordinary vitamin supplements). The other half received placebos that did not contain iron.

In short tests carried out at the end of the study period, the girls who had received the pills containing iron had higher scores in memorizing and verbal learning than those who had not received iron. It is both striking and troubling that a small reduction in blood levels of iron, a condition that is extremely common, can reduce learning capacity and memory in girls.

Endometriosis

Endometriosis is probably the most common cause of pelvic pain in women of reproductive age. Its frequency in infertile women ranges from 12 to 43 percent. The prevalence among fertile women is between 2 and 7 percent. The overall global rate of endometriosis in women of reproductive age is estimated to be about 10 percent. With the present world population of six billion, the United Nations estimates that there are one and a half billion women of reproductive age (age fifteen to forty-nine). Consequently, about one hundred fifty million women probably have endometriosis, whether or not it has been diagnosed. As the population grows, fertility declines, and the frequency of pelvic surgery including Caesarean section increases, the prevalence of endometriosis will certainly grow. The disease is now a major health problem for women and since curing endometriosis is difficult and recurrence is the rule rather than the exception, the situation is bound to worsen.

Endometriosis is a disease caused and routinely exacerbated by menstruation. The disease always manifests itself after the menarche and regresses at the menopause. In addition to causing severe pelvic pain during menstruation (dysmenorrhea) and in some cases, during sexual intercourse (dyspareunia), endometriosis is the principal cause of female infertility around the world, according to surveys carried out by the World Health Organization. The disease is caused by adhesion of fragments of the internal lining of the uterus, the endometrium, onto other organs and tissues in the abdominal or pelvic cavity. These endometrial cells or tissue fragments are carried into the pelvic cavity by menstrual blood which flows back into the fallopian tubes during menstruation. When this blood and the endometrial tissue it carries come into contact with scarred or exposed areas, some cells stick to the surface of pelvic organs such as the ruptured ovarian follicle or cysts, areas damaged following infection by sexually transmitted diseases, or by lesions resulting from abdominal surgery. Inflamed or infected areas are particularly susceptible to colonization by endometrial cells or fragments.

The endometriotic implants can grow and bleed cyclically just as the endometrial lining of the uterine cavity grows and bleeds, in response to the hormonal stimuli that determine the transformations taking place in the uterus during the menstrual cycle. They can proliferate and bleed wherever there are favorable conditions for the formation of cysts, such as the surface of the ovary. Endometriomas also attach to other organs, including the intestine, bladder, urethra, serous membrane surrounding the uterus, ovarian ligaments, peritoneal wall, diaphragm, and even the lungs.

The treatment of endometriosis can be surgical or medical. Most doctors consider surgery to be the primary choice, particularly if the growths are accessible with a laparoscope. The objective of the surgery is to remove as much of the endometriomal growth as possible. Sometimes this means removal of the entire affected organ. Medical treatment is initiated to inhibit menstruation and to promote the involution or atrophy of the endometriotic lesions. In young women, every effort should be made to preserve the woman's fertility whether the treatment is surgical or medical. Establishing a pregnancy effectively halts the disease process because when a woman is amenorrheic, as is the case during pregnancy, endometriosis does not manifest itself and usually does not progress. A definitive cure, however, has so far been elusive; women with endometriosis are always subject to recurrences.

In addition to the painful dysmenorrhea, endometriosis is a disorder that can cause considerable pain during intercourse (dyspareunia) and is a major cause of infertility. Depending on individual situations, the impact on marriages can be destructive. In cultures that hold fertility high on the list of requirements expected in a marriage, endometriosis can have a serious effect on the lives of women.

The devastating effect endometriosis can cause is illustrated by the following medical account of Marilyn Monroe's struggle with the disease. These facts have been drawn from documented biographies written by Donald Spoto and Anthony Sumners. From a medical viewpoint, I've also added my own interpretation of the impact her severe endometriosis had in contributing to many of the tragic circumstances of her life.

In considering Marilyn Monroe's battle with endometriosis, it is important to remember that until the 1960s, the ultimate recourse for controlling severe cases was to remove a woman's ovaries in order to put an end to the periodic stimulation of the endometrial tissue. Present-day laser surgery was not available and there were no other effective medical treatments. Thanks to progress in medicine, the diagnosis of the disease can now be made earlier, and the treatment, whether medical or surgical, is much more conservative and efficient. Not available during the years of Marilyn's affliction were the several forms of hormonal treatment, used now throughout the world. In spite of the seriousness of her endometriosis, Ms. Monroe refused to undergo the then-utilized surgery to remove her ovaries— most likely because she desperately wanted to become a mother. She endured the severe monthly pain by consuming greater and greater quantities of narcotics, ultimately leading to her death by overdose.

According to published biographical accounts of her life and in spite of her image as the ultimate sex symbol conveyed by Hollywood publicists, the actress's personal sexuality provided her little gratification or satisfaction. The painful dyspareunia characteristic of severe endometriosis made her resistant, tense, and apprehensive of intercourse. According to her biographers, Marilyn Monroe expressed her dissatisfaction with sex to her closest friends. By age twenty, already married for four years, Ms. Monroe complained of terrible cramps that complicated her career as a model, making it difficult for her to stand for long periods of time at photographic sessions. This symptom, along with the dysmenorrhea and dyspareunia that plagued her, reveals that she began suffering from advanced endometriosis at a young age.

In 1952 in Hollywood, while making the picture *Monkey Business* with Cary Grant, Marilyn Monroe had such severe abdominal pains that filming had to be stopped. Dr. Elliot Corday diagnosed appendicitis but she persuaded the doctor to delay the operation and for several days she was hospitalized, receiving antibiotic treatment. After a week, Marilyn returned to work without having undergone any surgery. The pain ascribed publicly to appendicitis was probably caused by endometriosis. After further weeks of suffering, Marilyn's publicist announced she *was* undergoing an appendectomy, carried out at the end of April. However, Dr. Marcus Rabwin, a general surgeon, brought in a gynecologist, Dr. Leon Krohn, to assist him with the surgery—a good clue that there was more than just an appendectomy being performed. In those days, "an appendectomy" would have been considered by Hollywood image makers as more acceptable for a young star, than surgery for "a woman's condition." After that first surgery, the gynecologist, Dr. Krohn, took over the treatment of the chronic menstrual problems of the enigmatic actress.

On November 7, 1954, Ms. Monroe had her second abdominal surgery at the Cedars of Lebanon Hospital. This surgery was described by gynecologist Krohn as "correction of a female disorder that had bothered her for years." Clarifying, he explained that he was referring to an operation to treat her "chronic endometriosis." This confirmed that when he had assisted in the appendectomy two years earlier, the presence of endometriosis had already been confirmed.

Marilyn Monroe and Arthur Miller were married in June 1956. She wanted to have a child but her endometriosis was probably the major reason she could not conceive, but there were also other possible reasons for her infertility. The continuous use and large quantity of analgesics and hypnotics, principally barbiturates taken to numb her pain probably interfered with ovulation. Her gynecologist, Leon Krohn, provided Marilyn with these prescription drugs without which she could not sleep. The fact that Dr. Krohn was always on the set while Marilyn was filming shows just how dependent the actress became on these powerful drugs.

In July 1957, an ecstatic Monroe learned that she was pregnant. It appeared that she had overcome her endometriosis but its physical effects remained a formidable obstacle to her happiness. Within a few days, in considerable pain, she was taken to Doctors Hospital in New York, where an ectopic pregnancy was diagnosed, most likely the result of endometriosis of the fallopian tube. She was operated on immediately and on that day lost not only the long-desired pregnancy, but also the fallopian tube where the ectopic implantation had taken place.

The following year, Marilyn Monroe again became pregnant. Sadly, she had a miscarriage before completing three months of pregnancy. Marilyn blamed herself because of the barbiturates she was taking and went into a period of depression. The sedatives that she had been taking since 1953 also possibly contributed to her depression.

On June 25, 1958, Ms. Monroe was hospitalized at the Lenox Hill Hospital in New York for a fourth surgical intervention. The operation was for the removal of endometriomas that were causing her "abnormally painful menstrual periods, severe bleeding and infertility."

In the summer of 1960, when Marilyn Monroe was filming *The Misfit* with Clark Gable, which would be her last picture, she was in constant agony with abdominal pain, which made even eating difficult. Before beginning each scene, she would be so ill that medical attention was necessary. With all the problems affecting her, she sought someone who would give her psychological and moral support. Thus began her relationship with Los Angeles psychoanalyst Dr. Ralph Greeson, to whom she became very attached, and who would be with the star to the last day of her life. Dr. Greeson recommended his colleague, Dr. Hyman Engelberg, to care for his famous patient's physical problems, and from then on, the pair of doctors worked to relieve Marilyn of her substantial burden of physical and mental problems. Engelberg was responsible for the continuous prescription of hypnotics that Marilyn required in order to be able to sleep. Tormented by persistent pain in the right side of her abdomen and severe attacks of indigestion—both probably consequences of endometriosis—it is also not surprising that Monroe became dependent on barbiturates. Without them, her mental and physical suffering would have become unbearable.

Marilyn Monroe and Arthur Miller announced their divorce in 1960. In May 1961, she was hospitalized by Leon Krohn in the Cedars of Lebanon Hospital for a fifth gynecological operation, this time to remove tissue damaged by endometriosis. She was thirty-five years old. A month later, Marilyn was operated on once again. The alleged reason was a cholecystectomy due to gallstones. But, drawn from medical reports, it is likely that the surgeon took advantage of the opportunity to continue the surgical efforts to remove endometriomal tissue from her pelvic and abdominal organs, an effort that now stretched over eight years and six operations.

According to friends, Marilyn had a whole pharmacy of prescription medications at home. The tranquilizers Valium and Librium, which went on the market at that time, were added to the analgesics, sedatives, and hypnotics that the actress used daily to rid herself of the pain caused by endometriosis and enabled her to sleep at night. Her health problems caused her to leave work at the film studio on numerous occasions or to demand last-minute cancellations of a scheduled shoot. Ultimately, this led to her dismissal by Fox Studios.

Life took a turn for the better for Marilyn in 1962. She and Joe DiMaggio, her husband of a previous marriage, announced their plans to re-marry, setting August 8 as the date. The event was anticipated happily by both of them and by their fans. She was also re-hired by her studio with a major salary increase. While she was preparing for the wedding, Ms. Monroe continued to suffer from the pelvic pain that tormented her endlessly. On July 21, she was hospitalized at Cedars of Lebanon Hospital for yet another surgery, her seventh, to remove hemorrhagic tissue caused by endometriosis.

Home from the hospital, on the first of August, Marilyn phoned Leon Krohn, who had treated her endometriosis since her first operation in 1952, and invited him for dinner at her house. But later in the day, she called to cancel the dinner, promising to phone again in a few days. Marilyn awoke early in a good mood on Friday, August 3, visited the office of her psychoanalyst, Dr. Greeson, shopped for items for her wedding reception, and returned home to meet Dr. Hyman Engelberg. He gave her a pain-killing injection and a prescription for twenty-five capsules of Nembutal® to be used with chloral hydrate. On August 4, Marilyn stayed home, taking delivery of items she had ordered for the forthcoming wedding. In the afternoon, she received a visit from Dr. Greeson, who left around 9 P.M. Marilyn was on the phone with several friends during the rest of the evening. When she failed to answer a return call, the caller became alarmed and alerted her lawyer, Milton Rudin.

It was Dr. Greeson, accompanied by Milton Rudin, who found the actress dead at midnight. The high quantity of sodium pentobarbital (Nembutal) found in her liver was practically twice the blood level, and the concentration of chloral hydrate in her blood was greater than that of Nembutal. There was no trace of narcotics found either in the stomach or in the duodenum, but the colon was found to be congested and of a purplish color, suggestive of rectal administration of chloral hydrate and barbiturates.

It is probable that Marilyn Monroe's death, caused by an overdose of prescribed narcotics, was accidental. One cannot escape the conclusion that her endometriosis was a determining factor in the drug dependency that made her accidental death predictable.

Oral contraceptive pills had appeared in 1960 and could have been used to suppress her menstruations as a treatment for endometriosis, but there is no record that this approach had ever been attempted for Ms. Monroe. Actually, it would have been very unusual for the physicians treating her to prescribe the pill for this purpose because by then no studies had been done on the use of the new oral contraceptive for the treatment of endometriosis. And, of course, it was a period in her life when she hoped to have a baby. There was also concern in those early years, later proved to be unfounded, that the use of the pill could delay subsequent fertility.

Ironically, Dr. Edward T. Tyler, a physician and fertility expert who pioneered the development of oral contraceptives and understood its potential use in gynecological disorders, practiced in nearby Westwood, and had many Hollywood stars among his patients. Marilyn Monroe was not one of them. The injectable hormone, DepoProvera®, which inhibits ovulation and menstruation, was discovered a year after Marilyn's death. Other products to treat endometriosis, such as Danazol® and Gestrinone®, were introduced for use in the 1970s and '80s.

Marilyn Monroe was a victim of a disease, which, at the time she required help, could only be efficiently treated by removal of the ovaries, an operation that, if carried out, would have deprived her of the innate femininity that she came to epitomize. Maintaining her functional ovaries resulted in inevitable menstrual cycles, which contributed to spreading the endometriosis and causing the chronic pelvic pain that became unbearably aggravated during menstruation and during sexual intercourse. Endometriosis also denied her the ability to have children, which she desperately wanted. Just as Niobe of the Greek legend, it was difficult for Marilyn Monroe to accept that her fame and adulation could not shield her from being deprived of the feminine pleasures and satisfactions that were so easily and naturally enjoyed by other women.

It was not endometriosis that took the life of Marilyn Monroe but it certainly contributed substantially to her enormous mental and physical suffering, leading to her dependence on the pain-killing drugs which ultimately killed her.

Endometriosis, anemia, premenstrual syndrome, dysmenorrhea and other menstrual cycle–related diseases affect a large number of women. These disorders need not be considered an inevitable part of "the curse." They are a serious enough health threat to constitute the main reasons why women seek gynecological care.

6

∽

Natural Suppression of Menstruation

Menstrual cycles enter the lives of most women when they are about thirteen, as they reach the menarche, and end when the menopause is complete, around forty-five to fifty years of age. At the beginning and end of the span they may experience irregular cycles (oligomenorrhea). During the reproductive years, usually considered to be fifteen to forty-five, they often stop menstruating naturally, due to pregnancy and breast-feeding. With high fertility and long periods of lactation, therefore, the number of times that a woman actually experiences menstrual cycles can be dramatically curtailed. For many women in developing countries where most of the world's population lives, this pattern of frequent and long periods of menstrual suppression accurately describes their menstruation history. In any given month around the globe, because of the natural circumstances of age, pregnancy, and breast-feeding, there are certainly more women not menstruating than there are menstruating. Moreover, there is substantial evidence that exercise and diet can further reduce the number of menstrual periods a woman has in her lifetime.

Pregnancy

Once the menarche is established, pregnancy is the most common way for a normal woman to stop menstruating. Obviously, many women who suffer from menstruation-related problems are not prepared to become pregnant and have a baby. However, if a woman wishes to become pregnant it is incidentally an excellent means for alleviating some menstruation-related problems. Doctors know, for example, that for some patients with endometriosis, nine menstruation-free months of pregnancy would be effective therapy. During pregnancy, both ovulation and menstruation are suppressed. Any bleeding that may occur is considered abnormal and an indication of a potential problem with the ongoing pregnancy. When a woman makes the choice to have a child, the possible benefit to her health that a pregnancy can have may not be a significant reason for her decision. Nevertheless, women whose health would benefit from suspending their periods gain an incidental advantage from their pregnancy, just as women should avoid pregnancy when their health or life would be at risk.

Pseudo-Pregnancy

Pseudo-pregnancy or pseudocyesis is a condition that imitates gestation even though there is no actual pregnancy. It is imaginary pregnancy. Pseudocyesis is usually observed in women near the menopause or in young women who intensely desire pregnancy. Some specialists consider it an organic disease, while others interpret it as a psychological manifestation of an unfulfilled desire. Pseudocyesis is more common in societies that place high expectations of childbearing in marriage. In the United States, obstetricians can go through their entire professional careers without seeing a case. When pseudocyesis occurs in the earlier years of life, the menses do not as a rule disappear, but may become irregular. Older women may have long periods of anovulation, free from menstruation. Psychotic patients may persist for years in the delusion that they are pregnant, remaining free of menstruation during the entire time. It is difficult to persuade these women that they are not pregnant.

Pseudo-pregnant women have many of the subjective symptoms of pregnancy. There is a considerable increase in the size of the abdomen, caused by the deposition of fat or the accumulation of abdominal fluid. The increase in size of the abdomen can be as large as that of a full-term pregnancy. Pregnancy-like changes occur in the breasts including enlargement, the appearance of secretion, and increased pigmentation of the nipples. The majority of cases experience all the symptoms of morning sickness. Contractions of the muscles of the abdominal wall simulate fetal movements. From an endocrine point of view, the condition is characterized by a simultaneous and sustained rise in the ovulatory hormone, LH, and in prolactin.

Lactation

During lactation, ovulation inhibition is caused by a rise in the level of prolactin, a hormone produced by the pituitary gland. As prolactin secretion increases, the release of the pituitary's gonad-stimulating hormones, LH and FSH, decreases. This stops ovulation from occurring. Ovarian production of estradiol is also reduced to extremely low levels. In order for breast-feeding to inhibit ovulation, it has to be practiced on demand, whenever the baby requires feeding, day and night. When the infant is breast-fed exclusively, without supplementary feeding, the levels of prolactin remain high, and ovulation is blocked through the suppression of hormone production both at the pituitary level and at the ovarian level. This is because the neural stimulus caused by suckling suppresses the normal pattern of secretion of the gonadotropin-releasing hormone (GnRH or LHRH) and consequently LH itself. Without LH, ovarian follicles do not mature, estrogen production remains low, and ovulation does not occur. When the stimulus of breast-feeding ceases or diminishes, the pulsatile patterns of GnRH and LH secretion return to normal, the stimulated follicle grows again, producing estrogen, and these events lead to ovulation.

The inhibition of ovulation and menstruation caused by breast-feeding is very efficient in the first six months after delivery. In the following months, 50 percent of women start ovulating again, even when they are still breast-feeding on demand, because other food is usually given to the infant during this period. However, anthropologists report that some tribal women indigenous to South America breast-feed their children for as long as four years and that ovulation can be suppressed during the entire time. Women of the Dogon culture of West African farming villages nurse their children for almost two years. According to Strassmann these women have an average of about 110 menstrual periods in a lifetime, in contrast to the 400 experienced by women in industrialized countries. If this is so, apparently the children suckling stimulation maintains a high level of prolactin for these many years.

Ovulation suppression by lactation is the basis of a method called "LAM" (Lactational Amenorrhea Method) used in family planning programs. Pregnancy prevention during the lactational period is considered the most efficient natural method of birth control and, globally, probably contributes toward delaying pregnancies more often than all other methods combined. According to anthropologist R. B. Lee, who studied the !Kung San, a nomadic people who live in Africa, the spacing of four or more years between children of these hunter-gatherers is a result of lactation. !Kung women begin to menstruate at sixteen or seventeen years of age. Nearly seven out of ten marry before their first menstrual period. Most of the others marry at menarche. Seventy percent of !Kung wives have their first child by twenty-two years of age. Although they have an average of only four children during their reproductive life, each child is breast-fed for many years. About 50 percent of the !Kung women have their second child approximately four years after the first, while 25 percent have their second child three years after the first. When the !Kung become sedentary, the interval between children reduces because maternal fat reserves increase, hastening the return of ovulation.

Physical Exercise

Menstruation may be suppressed in young women who exercise regularly over a long period of time. The phenomenon is frequently experienced by runners, ballet dancers, gymnasts, weight-lifters, skaters, and even swimmers. Many physiological changes occur with exercise, including loss of body fat and the production of endorphins, natural opioids that reach brain receptors. One effect of endorphins is to inhibit the production of LH, the ovulatory hormone produced by the pituitary gland. With the subsequent inhibition of ovarian follicle development and ovulation, there is an automatic reduction in estrogen production by the ovary. Ovulation suppression, therefore, is linked to exercise through loss of body fat and the inhibiting action of endorphins on luteinizing hormone production by the pituitary. Since the production of other pituitary hormones may be affected also, women with exercise-induced amenorrhea should seek medical supervision.

Some sports physiologists believe that physical and psychic stress and the subsequent rise in the production of cortisone, the stress hormone, also play a role in inhibiting ovulation in athletes, causing oligomenorrhea (reduction in frequency of menstruation) or amenorrhea (absence of menstruation). In one important study, menstruation-related information was obtained from a group of four hundred seventy-five Nigerian athletes. Regular menstrual cycles were recorded in only 25 percent of them. The athletes who menstruated least were the marathon runners and soccer and basketball players.

Another study compared runners who menstruated regularly and runners who did not menstruate. The principal difference between the two groups was the distance ran during training sessions. Women who put in an average of twenty-five miles of training a week continued to menstruate, while those who averaged over forty miles a week were often amenorrheic. Estrogen levels in the women athletes who did not menstruate fell to almost one-third the level found in athletes with normal menstruation. Accompanying the low estrogen values of non-menstruating athletes is a significant reduction in bone density of the lumbar verte- brae. In this and in other studies, no calcium loss in the long bones such as the femur and the radius was observed. There are data to suggest that the reduction in vertebral bone density may be associated more with loss of weight than with amenorrhea. A study done at a Harvard Medical School hospital revealed that amenorrheic athletes who do not experience weight loss retain normal bone density, while non-athletes have significant bone loss associated with amenorrhea resulting from weight-loss itself. When there is bone loss among athletes, a possible contributing factor may be the elevated levels of cortisol since this adrenal hor- mone is around 50 percent higher in women athletes who do not menstruate than in those who do menstruate.

Calcium loss from the vertebrae and the risk of osteo- porosis in athletes is counter-intuitive because physical ex- ercise is considered a principal means for preventing and combating osteoporosis, while immobility and lack of ex- ercise is thought to be a contributing factor. In addition, studies show that there is a direct correlation between the amount of exercise done by amenorrheic athletes and den- sity in the long bones of the extremities. Despite the re- duction in bone density in the vertebrae, women athletes maintain greater bone density than non-athletes after men- opause. This indicates that, over time, women athletes do not suffer the calcium loss observed in non-athletes. Related observations in male athletes reveal that heavily perspiring basketball players lose calcium, resulting in a significant re- duction in bone density. Bone density returns to normal in these men following one year of calcium supplementation.

In a 1995 study carried out at Oregon State University, it was observed that gymnasts maintain greater bone den- sity than runners, despite a similar prevalence of amenorrhea and irregular menstruation. In addition, gymnasts begin menstruating later (average 16.2 years) than runners (average 14.4 years) and individuals who did not do any physical exercise (13.0 years). The prevalence of oligomenorrhea (infrequent menstruation) and amenorrhea is 47 percent for gymnasts, 30 percent for runners and near zero for non-athletes. Bone density of lumbar vertebrae of gymnasts is greater than the bone density of non-athletes while that of runners is less than that of controls. Bone density of the cervical vertebrae of gymnasts is also greater than that of non-athletes who menstruate regularly and, in turn, have greater bone density than that of runners.

These observations lead to the conclusion that gymnasts who exercise their entire bodies, even though they become amenorrheic, have an increase, not decrease, in density of the entire skeleton. This certainly helps to prevent osteoporosis later in life. Tennis players and weight lifters derive the same benefit from their participation in the sport of their choice. In a study carried out in older athletes who had exercised vigorously at least three times a week for eight or more months of the year for a minimum of three years, it was found that vertebral bone density was significantly higher in tennis players. Lumbar vertebral bone density of older athletes, between fifty-five and seventy-five years of age, was the same as in younger athletes.

Another study carried out at the University of Arizona found that weight-lifting increases bone density in lumbar vertebrae of pre-menopausal women between twenty-eight and thirty-nine years of age. At the end of one year, the increase was over 2 percent. Increase in the density of the femur at twelve months was over 1 percent and at eighteen months this increase reached 2 percent.

Another group of athletes who respond to exercise differently from runners are swimmers. They experience a delay in the onset of menstruation, as well as amenorrhea, as runners do. But, contrary to runners, estrogen levels remain high, both in those who begin swimming training before menarche and in those who begin to swim after menarche. Eighty-two percent of swimmers encounter amenorrhea or menstrual irregularity. This is about double the percentage in the control group. In addition, the duration of episodes of amenorrhea is sixteen months in swimmers, compared to only four months in the controls. From an endocrine point of view, the alterations found in swimmers were a rise in androgens, dihydroepiandrosterone (DHEA), and androstenedione, but not in testosterone.

This information demonstrates that it is not simple to stop menstruating deliberately by practicing physical exercise. The type of training involved in these studies demands discipline, perseverance, determination, and good health. Those who are willing to undertake the conscientious practice of exercise, whether sport or dance, before the first menstrual period, can delay the onset of the menarche for several years. For each year of exercise, the onset of menstruation is delayed for an average of five months. Adolescents who have a delay of menarche caused by exercise will have irregular cycles or amenorrhea if they continue to exercise at the same level of intensity.

For the suppression of menstrual periods to occur in women who menstruate regularly and who wish to do this by running, it would be necessary to exceed twenty-five miles weekly. This means running over three miles a day, every day of the week. For runners who manage to remain amenorrheic, it is wise to maintain a reasonable level of estrogen to prevent possible bone loss. In well-monitored women, it is necessary to provide a progestin only if a thickening of the endometrium is observed by ultrasound examination. In view of the popularity of running, doctors are frequently consulted regarding how to protect women runners against osteoporosis. In a questionnaire given to family doctors and sports specialists, almost all who answered agreed with the use of estrogenic hormones (92 percent) and with calcium supplementation (87 percent). An increase in caloric intake was suggested by 64 percent while a reduction in exercise level was the choice of 57 percent.

It is clear that those who wish to choose the sport most adequate for suppressing menstruation without worry about calcium loss should choose gymnastics or swimming. Other good options are tennis and weight-bearing routines. It is also possible to find combinations of sports, such as tennis with dance, gymnastics with running. There is no evidence that alterations to the menstrual cycle induced by physical exercise harm the reproductive system, but it is obvious that if a woman wishes to become pregnant she will have to reduce the level or the intensity of her exercise so that she will start ovulating again. Medical supervision is indispensable to avoid the risk of health problems that would outweigh possible benefits of menstrual suppression. Careful monitoring of thyroid function and other endocrine parameters is essential.

7

∞

Medical Suppression of Menstruation

Substantial health benefits can be derived from adopting menstruation suppression as standard practice. The most radical way to end menstruation irreversibly is to surgically remove a woman's ovaries (oophorectomy or ovariectomy) and/or uterus (hysterectomy). Obviously, this is not an option for women who wish to preserve their fertility. However, modern medicine can now achieve the same result without drastic surgery and with the assurance of reversibility that allows a woman to be confident that she can maintain her reproductive potential.

This therapy began with the advent of the oral contraceptive pill in the early 1960s. When this ovulation-inhibiting medication was developed and introduced for use in birth control, it was less widely publicized that with this drug it was possible for women to control their own menstruation. Understandably, doctors may have been reluctant to advise normal, healthy women to continuously take a drug with which they had little experience. But as its use has grown, it is has been found that the health benefits outweigh the risks. Women should have the information to consider the use of ovulation-suppressing hormone pills without cyclical interruption in order to prevent menstruation. The strategy to market "the pill" to mimic menstruation was primarily a marketing decision. There was no scientific or medical basis to assume that intermittent use of the new product would be better or safer than continuous use. Not long after the pill became available, we discovered in Brazil that the injectable progestin medroxyprogesterone acetate (MPA), trade named DepoProvera®, can suppress ovulation and menstruation for months at a time, and that women can safely be amenorrheic by simply taking four injections a year. Several other progestins, administered either orally or vaginally, can achieve the same purpose. Other options are a system of sub-dermal capsules or a medicated intra-uterine system that can induce amenorrhea in some women for several years. As a medical substitute for removal of the ovaries, analogues of peptide hormones produced in the brain can be used, but this produces all the symptoms of menopause unless used simultaneously with steroid hormone add-back therapy.

Hysterectomy

The first hysterectomy was carried out in 1822. While some of the operations done currently are life-saving (to cure cancer or stop hemorrhage), the great majority are carried out for the relief of menstrual cycle–related symptoms, usually excessive bleeding (menorrhagia). The operation has become extremely safe since it was first carried out in the last century. However, its predominant place in therapy has been seriously challenged in recent years as alternative treatments have appeared.

Hysterectomy is the most radical among the various means to stop menstruation. Removing the uterus guarantees the irreversible end of menstrual bleeding and the accompanying dysmenorrhea. What hysterectomy alone does not solve is the problem of premenstrual tension, which will continue to plague the woman until menopause, when ovarian function ceases and with it, the hormonal fluctuations responsible for the premenstrual syndrome.

For this reason, hysterectomy can be considered as a solution for serious complications associated with the menstrual period itself, such as uncontrolled bleeding and incessant severe cramps. The most frequent indications are myomas or fibromas, extreme endometrial growth (hyperplasia or polyps), some cases of endometriosis, particularly when the disease involves the uterus itself (called adeno-myosis), excessive bleeding caused by defects in the mechanism of blood coagulation, and anemia. Prolonged menstrual blood loss due to coagulation defects in patients undergoing kidney dialysis can make hysterectomy imperative.

In the United States, it is not uncommon for women who have already completed their families to elect to undergo hysterectomy in order to rid themselves of a potential cause of uterine problems that are more frequent in premenopause, or simply to put an end to menstruation. Some authors have expressed the view that the frequency of hysterectomy represents an overuse of this surgery.

More than fifteen million hysterectomies were done in the United States between 1965 and 1984. Dr. I. K. Strausz, Professor of Obstetrics and Gynecology at the New York Medical College, wrote a book in 1994 for women readers with the provocative title *You Don't Need a Hysterectomy*. In this book, he condemns the ease with which American women undergo hysterectomies, presenting a long list of possible complications of hysterectomy which, Dr. Strausz believes, should make the operation the last option to be considered by women who wish to rid themselves of menstruation. His list includes complications associated with any operation, such as anesthesia risks, along with emotional consequences, surgical lesions, adhesions, blood transfusions, thrombosis, incisional hernia, intestinal obstruction, sexual difficulties, and premature menopause. Strausz also contends that the mortality rate associated with the operation is slightly higher than one-tenth of 1 percent, or more than one in one thousand women. The argument that deserves special attention is the possible initiation of menopause in relatively young women.

Removal of the uterus can change ovarian function because of modifications in blood circulation between the two ovaries and the uterus. In some women, the intervention can indeed bring on an early menopause. To avoid the consequences of an early menopause, women who undergo hysterectomy are advised to begin hormone replacement therapy with estrogen earlier than others. But these women have the advantage of being able to do so without requiring the progestin complement which is recommended for those women who have a uterus. Without a uterus, some women report a loss of a sense of purpose, or may be made to feel this loss by uncaring or unsupportive partners. This can result in severe damage to a couple's relationship. Some men and women believe that the presence of the uterus is necessary for women to have satisfying sexual experiences. In spite of these perceived disadvantages, in recent years some women have opted for elective hysterectomy as a preventive measure when they discover that they have genetic risk factors for endometrial cancer.

Endometrial Resection

Less radical than hysterectomy for ending menstrual bleeding, endometrial resection is the removal of the internal lining of the uterus, the endometrium, with the help of a special instrument called a hysteroscope. This is inserted into the uterus through the vagina and cervix. Since menstrual bleeding is a result of the collapse of the spiral arteries which nourish the endometrium, the removal of the cell layer containing these blood vessels by electric cauterization or laser puts an end to periodic menstrual bleeding.

The method has become very popular in recent years because it eliminates the part of the uterus responsible for excessive bleeding. The procedure can be carried out under general, regional, or local anesthesia and normally takes less than thirty minutes. Unfortunately, ablation or resection of the endometrium does not always result in complete suppression of menstruation because the endometrium can regenerate if a sufficient portion of the cells is left undisturbed. Complete suppression is achieved in 25 to 60 percent of cases. In the remaining cases, however, a significant reduction in blood loss is achieved. More than 80 percent of women who undergo endometrial ablation express satisfaction with the procedure. The blood loss which serves as an indication for this type of procedure was calculated in one Australian study as being around one hundred and sixty milliliters per cycle. Six months after the operation, the average blood loss was reduced to less than two milliliters per cycle. The pain associated with extensive menstrual bleeding generally disappears after endometrial ablation. However, premenstrual tension continues unaltered in the majority of patients, just as it does following hysterectomy without removal of the ovaries.

Endometrial ablation, although a less serious procedure than hysterectomy, can also result in complications. The uterus can be perforated and damage to other pelvic organs, such as the intestine and the bladder, can result from accidental contact with the electrodes used for the endometrial ablation. In experienced hands these incidents, which can also happen during other laparoscopic procedures, are minimized.

Endometrial ablation is less costly than hysterectomy, is considerably less invasive, and requires less time for hospitalization and recovery. Both cost and time in the hospital are reduced about 50 percent. Time required for the woman to return to normal activities, post-operatively, is substantially shortened.

Although endometrial ablation greatly reduces a woman's chance of ever becoming pregnant, risk of a pregnancy occurring after the operation still exists. Ectopic pregnancy in the fallopian tubes, for example, can occur at the same rate as in women who have not had the operation. Intra-uterine pregnancy can also occur although this is quite rare in women who have had endometrial ablation.

Endometrial ablation does not free women from the risk of developing cancer in the remnants of the endometrium, so hormone replacement therapy, when required, should always include a progestin.

Oophorectomy (Ovariectomy)

Since menstruation and the premenstrual syndrome are consequences of the cyclical production of hormones by the ovaries, women without ovarian function neither menstruate nor suffer from premenstrual tension. Dr. R. Frank reported in 1931 that X-ray ablation of the ovaries resulted in the disappearance not only of menstruation but also of the characteristic symptoms of the premenstrual syndrome. The major limitation of Frank's approach was the premature menopause which is unavoidable if ovarian function is terminated and hormone replacement is not initiated. When he carried out his studies nearly seventy years ago, the concept and means for add-back hormonal therapy had not yet emerged. Recently, Frank's original proposal was re-evaluated and the surgical removal of the ovaries began to be considered when all other therapeutic approaches prove to be unsuccessful for the treatment of severe cases of menstrual cycle–related disorders, including premenstrual syndrome. In these cases, the uterus is removed together with the ovaries. Dr. Allison Case and Dr. Robert Reid of the Department of Obstetrics and Gynaecology of Queen's University in Kingston, Ontario published a review article in 1998 covering over one hundred and fifty publications in peer-reviewed scientific journals on the subject of menstrual cycle–related medical disorders. They conclude that in certain cases when medical conditions are seriously exacerbated during the menstrual cycle, "consideration of hysterectomy and bilateral oophorectomy with ongoing estrogen replacement therapy is appropriate."

Oral Contraceptives

Less drastic than surgical methods, the use of the oral contraceptive pill can be the most accessible solution for women who wish to stop menstruating and, at the same time, to rid themselves of premenstrual symptoms. Since both menstruation and the symptoms preceding it are a result of the cyclical production of ovarian hormones, the inhibition of this function results in the disappearance of menstruation. It is an option that should be explained to women who suffer from menstrual problems. Long-term ovulation inhibition can be maintained for months or even years, by the continuous use of contraceptive pills taken orally. In many cases of dysmenorrhea in young women, the classical intermittent use of contraceptive pills (twenty-one days per month) can solve the problem as the bleeding caused by the discontinuation of the pill often occurs without pain. However, when the pain continues at the same intensity, continuous use of the pill can solve the problem by preventing the bleeding entirely.

The Vaginal Contraceptive Pill

The same result, including the disappearance of menstruation and the symptoms of premenstrual syndrome, can be obtained by using the contraceptive pill vaginally instead of orally. Women with premenstrual syndrome symptoms, including insomnia, nervousness, pelvic pain, and headache, have been maintained in amenorrhea, asymptomatic for periods longer than five years by prescribing the pill vaginally on an uninterrupted daily basis. Continuous use appears to increase the efficacy of the pill as compared to intermittent use. An advantage of using the pill vaginally is that it can reduce the frequency or severity of gastrointestinal side effects that some women experience when taking the same pill orally. Although there is presently no contraceptive pill specifically formulated for vaginal use in the U.S. market, conventional oral contraceptive products can be used. Pharmaceutical companies should turn their attention to designing a tablet or other delivery system that would optimize the vaginal route of administration. The first such product, in fact, is being marketed by a company in Brazil.

Injectable Contraceptives (MPA)

The injectable contraceptive ideal for suppressing menstruation is medroxyprogesterone acetate (MPA), which is marketed as DepoProvera®. MPA has prolonged action as an ovulation inhibitor. A dose of fifty milligrams inhibits ovulation for one month, one hundred and fifty milligrams inhibits ovulation for three months, and a dose of four hundred milligrams inhibits ovulation for six months. One gram will inhibit ovulation for one year. The effect is reversible and can be used in young women who wish to preserve their fertility. The success of MPA in suppressing menstruation is higher than 70 percent and its contraceptive efficacy is one of the highest of all contraceptive methods, similar to the rate obtained with contraceptive surgery (tubal ligation). Its low cost makes MPA widely accessible. The occurrence of occasional bleeding, spotting, or persistent staining in some users is the principal drawback of MPA when used to suppress ovulation. When it is used for contraception, the large percentage of women who become amenorrheic is a drawback to continued use unless users are well-informed to expect this result and its benefits.

Monthly injectable contraceptives consisting of a progestin and estrogen were developed in order to provide an injectable contraceptive method for women who choose to preserve periodic bleeding. For this reason, this method cannot be used to induce amenorrhea. However, its use by patients who have no complaints associated with the actual bleeding can provide relief from the symptoms of premenstrual syndrome.

Contraceptive Implants

Subdermal implants containing progestins such as those used in contraceptive pills constitute a modern method of contraception that can also be used to inhibit ovulation and consequently menstruation. The first of these products to be introduced onto the market, Norplant®, consists of a set of six soft, tubular capsules of Silastic® containing the progestin levonorgestrel. There is now a second version of this product that has the same effectiveness and requires only two elongated inserts. Levonorgestrel is the active component of a large number of contraceptive products marketed throughout the world. In the aggregate, the sale of these products makes levonorgestrel the most widely used progestin in the world's contraceptive market. The subcutaneous insertion of Norplant® capsules is usually done, following topical anesthesia, in the upper arm. The Norplant® system is available in the United States and various European countries and is widely used in Asia. Millions of women have used it for contraception since it was first approved for use in Europe in the 1980s and in the United States in 1991.

The contraceptive effect of Norplant® can be prolonged for more than five years but its suppressive effect on ovulation and menstruation can be relied upon primarily in the first year. In most patients, the use of Norplant® results in a bleeding pattern that does not fulfill the objective of inhibiting ovulation and menstruation.

There are other sub-dermal contraceptive implant systems that are long-acting and can be used for suppression of ovulation and menstruation. The most advanced is called Implanon®. It consists of a single capsule made of ethyl vinyl acetate (EVA), not Silastic®. Implanon®, like Norplant®, contains a progestin used extensively as an oral contraceptive (3-ketodesorgestrel). It can last for three years as a contraceptive and works primarily by suppressing ovulation. After the first three months of use, the incidence of amenorrhea among women using Implanon® is about 35 percent for the remainder of the first year, remains at about this percentage during the second year, and gradually declines thereafter.

Surplant® consists of a single capsule which provides contraception for one year and which can be renewed for as long as the patient desires. More than one half of the women who use Uniplant® bleed regularly as if they were menstruating. To suppress ovulation, two, or even three, Surplant® capsules can be effective. For example, forty-six out of one hundred cycles proved to be anovulatory when women used two capsules of Uniplant®. Another compound which can be used to suppress ovulation and menstruation in implant form is a steroid referred to as ST-1435, the code name assigned to it when it was first synthesized by chemists at the Merck Company, in Germany. Now it is also called Nesterone® in the United States and Elcometrine® in Brazil. It will first enter the Brazilian market as a treatment for endometriosis and for contraception in lactating women. It is particularly suitable for this purpose because the compound is not active when taken orally, so that if there is any present in the mother's milk, the suckling baby is protected from its biological effects. A single implant containing ST-1435 provides contraceptive protection by inhibiting ovulation in all users. Menstruation suppression therefore occurs in all cases. However, occasional bleeding occurs in 50 percent of patients. The duration of effect of one capsule is six months, but insertion can be repeated at the end of each six-month period.

Medicated Intrauterine System (IUS)

Presently, there is only one IUS that may be suitable for medical suppression of menstruation. This is marketed in Europe as Mirena®, where it is sold as a contraceptive and may soon be available in the United States and elsewhere. Like Norplant®, this method utilizes levonorgestrel as the progestin for achieving the contraceptive effect. The Mirena® system results in considerably less unintended bleeding and, used continuously, establishes amenorrhea in a large percentage of users.

Risk Analysis
of Hormonal Suppression of Menstruation

It is important to evaluate whether long-term use of ovulation-suppressing hormones introduces risks that could offset some of the benefits of menstruation reduction or elimination. Most evidence is based on the extensive experience with the use of hormonal contraception, the pill, which can serve as an ovulation inhibitor. The consensus of expert opinion after nearly four decades of use of the pill favors the view that this medication carries with it impressive health benefits in several areas. In addition to the ability to alleviate menstrual cycle–related disorders such as endometriosis and functional ovarian cysts, it is associated with a reduced risk of ovarian and endometrial cancer and decreased rates of benign tumors of the breast and uterus. It protects the cardiovascular system against some types of life-threatening disease, and it maintains healthy bone density as women grow older and approach menopause.

Steroid hormone contraceptives have been available since the 1960s and are now used by more than one hundred million women worldwide. In the United States alone there are over sixteen million users. Reports linking the original pill with cardiovascular side effects (venous thrombosis) appeared soon after these products were first marketed. Since then a major drop in the estrogen and progestin levels have made oral contraceptives safer and broadened the spectrum of their beneficial effects. The original contraceptive pill contained one hundred and fifty micrograms of estrogen. Today's pill contains twenty to fifty micrograms. Progestin content of the early pill was about ten milligrams. Now the products contain about one milligram. As characterized in an October 1998 *New York Times* article, this is "not your mother's birth control pill." When the first oral contraceptives came out, there was a scare regarding increased risk of thrombophlebitis and other types of venous thrombosis.

Since then, many epidemiological studies have investigated whether users of the pill are at increased risk of cardiovascular disease. In general, women of reproductive age enjoy a very low risk of vascular diseases (stroke, heart attack, and venous thromboembolism). Any additional cardiovascular disease incidence or mortality attributable to oral contraceptives has been shown to be insignificant if users do not smoke or lack other risk factors. Studying all available information, a World Health Organization scientific panel concluded in 1998 that there is no substantive evidence of increased risk of myocardial infarction (heart attack) among users of combined oral contraceptives, compared with women who never have used them.

The risk of suffering a stroke while taking the pill is age-related, and also very much dependent on whether the woman smokes. There are two main types of strokes: occlusion of a blood vessel in the brain (ischemic stroke) and bleeding in the brain from a blood vessel (hemorrhagic stroke). The reported estimates of relative risk of ischemic stroke associated with the use of oral contraceptives have steadily decreased since the earliest epidemiological linkage was made. This declining risk is due to the use of low-dose hormonal contraceptives (with less than fifty micrograms of estrogen). When using these products, women who do not smoke and do not have high blood pressure have a minimally increased chance of ischemic stroke than non-users. Age appears to be a pivotal factor. The risk among users of combined oral contraceptives who are over age thirty-five is more than among those who are under thirty-five. For all women and particularly for women over thirty-five, smoking or high blood pressure are much more potent risk factors than is use of the pill. The risk of hemorrhagic stroke in women who smoke is up to twice that in non-smokers; in women who are smokers and users of combined oral contraceptives, the risk is increased considerably. In the absence of other risk factors, there is no evidence that either the estrogen or the progestin constituent of combined oral contraceptives alters the risk of hemorrhagic stroke. In other words, non-smoking women under thirty-five years of age with normal blood pressure do not incur an increased risk of hemorrhagic stroke with use of combined oral contraceptives.

The association of oral contraceptive use and venous thromboembolism, including events of deep venous thrombosis and related blood clots in the lung, has been widely studied over the years. It is a complex situation because the composition of oral contraceptives has changed constantly both in the content of estrogen and progestin, and in the nature of the progestin. So-called first-generation pills usually contained greater than fifty micrograms of estrogen; most of these are no longer being marketed. Second-generation pills contain less than fifty micrograms of estrogen and a familiar progestin such as norethindrone or levonorgestrel. Next came a new generation of pills utilizing progestins with less androgenicity. This third generation was rapidly replacing older formulations until a World Health Organization report in 1996 suggested that the new products were associated with a somewhat higher risk of venous thrombosis than earlier products. This created controversy about the safety of oral contraceptives in general and many women became frightened of the method. Since then, there have been excellent new analyses and new studies so that a clearer picture has emerged.

It is important to realize that all studies on the associations between oral contraceptives and cardiovascular disease are limited by the extreme rarity of these problems among young women. Early studies that followed the experience of large numbers of women over a period of many years only have data regarding older oral contraceptive formulations that are now little used, if at all. Nevertheless, there have been studies concentrating on newer formulations and they confirm that there is a detectable association between combination oral contraceptive use and venous thrombosis that correlates with the estrogen dose. This association has been the main motivation for oral contraceptives with lower estrogen dosages.

A huge study in the United Kingdom including observations on over a half million women of reproductive age found the rate of venous thrombosis to be about one per ten thousand women per year among women who were neither pregnant nor using oral contraceptives. The rates were about six per ten thousand women in those who were pregnant or post-partum and three per ten thousand in those using combined oral contraceptives. Thus, oral contraceptive use increases the risk slightly (from a very low baseline rate) but less so than pregnancy.

The rates of occurrence of all adverse cardiovascular events, including venous thromboembolism, in pregnancy and the post-partum period are four to six times higher than among pill users. Experts conclude that the difference in clinical importance among formulations with respect to adverse cardiovascular outcomes is minor and hard to detect because of the extremely low baseline incidence of these disorders among women of reproductive age. The absolute rates of venous thromboembolism among pill-users have been dropping steadily and appreciably since the oral contraceptives were introduced. The evidence shows that, in this respect, oral contraceptives on the market are safe and getting safer.

The discussion of the association of oral contraceptives and cancer focuses mainly on reproductive organ cancers. Ovarian cancer is the fourth leading cause of cancer deaths in women. It is fatal for almost 80 percent of women who develop it. A woman's chance of getting ovarian cancer decreases with an increase in her periods of anovulation, including the use of the pill. An important study carried out by the National Institutes of Health concluded that the use of oral contraceptives decreases the risk of ovarian cancer. This cancer risk decreases as the duration of contraceptive use increases, and the protective effect persists long after the woman ceases to use oral contraceptives.

Cancer of the uterine lining, the endometrium, is also a common disease. The risk of endometrial cancer in women who have used oral contraceptives for at least two years is about 40 percent less than among women who have never used combined oral contraceptives. The longer a woman uses the pill, the greater her protection against this cancer.

Breast cancer is the most frequently occurring reproductive organ cancer, so this is the association with hormonal contraception that, understandably, concerns most women. All told, there are over thirty studies on this subject. Some show no change in risk, others show a reduction in risk, and still others reveal an increase in risk. For example, a study in Sweden found that women who start using the pill at an early age and continue for at least three years slightly increase their risk of breast cancer. In the same study, older age groups showed no change in the rate of breast cancer. A recent World Health Organization study covering over fifty thousand women in many countries concluded that there is a small increase in the risk of breast cancer while women are taking the combined pill or if they have used the method during the past ten years. Benign breast disease, commonly called fibrocystic disease, is less likely to occur in women using oral contraceptives. This appears to be a progestin-related protection.

A study published in the *British Medical Journal* in January 1999 finally dispels fears that have lingered about the long-term safety of oral contraceptives since their use began forty years ago. The study involved forty-six thousand British women tracked for twenty-five years. The study shows no lasting ill effects from taking hormonal contraceptive pills for as long as ten years. Ten years after they stopped using the pill, the women's chances of dying from cancer, stroke, or other side effects were not increased over the chances of women who had never taken it. Significantly, most women in the study were taking pills of higher dose than the ones available today. This gives added assurance of long-term safety for today's young women who are just beginning to use the pill for contraception or for the hormonal suppression of menstruation.

Gestrinone® and Danazol®

Danazol® and Gestrinone® are synthetic steroid hormones that can be used as oral pills to suppress ovulation and menstruation. Although both products are recommended specifically for the treatment of endometriosis, they can be used in other conditions in which there is pain associated with menstruation and/or excessive bleeding. Although they act similarly, Gestrinone® has the advantage of being more potent in terms of potency per weight of drug. The quantity of Gestrinone® administered over one year corresponds to the amount of Danazol® administered in one day of treatment. In addition to requiring lower doses, Gestrinone® offers a more convenient schedule of administration and is far less costly. An important advantage of Gestrinone® is its effect on the endometrium, which becomes atrophic without causing menopausal symptoms. Gestrinone® can also be used in implant form with the same efficacy as in the oral form. Four implants of fifty milligrams each are required to assure an inhibiting effect on ovulation for one year.

Gonadotropin Releasing Hormone Analogues (LHRH)

These therapeutic agents are synthetic peptides (small proteins), which have the capacity to inhibit ovulation through an action at the level of the brain and the pituitary gland. There are two types of analogues: agonists which mimic the activity of the natural hormone (LHRH) and antagonists which compete and interfere with the natural hormone. The agonist analogues initially have a brief stimulating effect but with their continued use they deplete the pituitary gland's ability to produce LH, the ovulation-inducing hormone, and this results in inhibiting ovulation. The antagonist analogues block the natural hormonal action of LHRH by competing with it at the level of the pituitary gland where its natural action is to stimulate the release of the ovulation hormone, LH.

A limitation of these products is that they can only be administered by injection or by nasal spray; they are not active orally. The extended use of these analogues creates an artificial menopause, reproducing all the symptoms of the natural menopause, including the cessation of menstruation and of all its symptoms. This gives the woman immediate relief. The adverse effects of the induced menopause limits the medication's use, unless it is used with add-back estrogen therapy. One option is to provide an LHRH analogue together with the simultaneous use of implants of estradiol, which protect the patient against practically all the adverse effects of the menopause.

Doctors now have an array of medical methods to suppress menstruation, either permanently or reversibly. As a non-surgical substitute for ovariectomy, LHRH analogues have an added importance since experience has grown with their use along with the simultaneous administration of add-back hormone therapy.

Sulpiride

Sulpiride is an anti-depressant that causes a substantial increase in the secretion of prolactin, the principal hormone responsible for lactation. The rise in prolactin causes inhibition of the secretion of the hormones responsible for ovulation induction. Since ovulation does not occur, neither does menstruation and, for this reason, women who use anti-depressants containing sulpiride do not menstruate. Similar compounds can induce amenorrhea in the same way. Two hundred to three hundred milligrams of sulpiride daily results in amenorrhea that can be maintained for long periods. Since this is not an over-the-counter medication, it can only be obtained by prescription.

Alternative Medicine

The use of alternative medicine for all reasons is widespread in the United States. A 1993 publication claimed that one in three Americans use unconventional forms of medical care and they spend over ten billion dollars on these products and services. Many "cures" come from the traditional medicines of other countries, usually derived from botanicals or plant products. As dietary supplements, they are not regulated by the Food and Drug Administration and therefore do not have to provide evidence establishing effectiveness and safety.

American women are familiar with drugstore products for alleviating menstrual symptoms, such as Lydia Pinkham's Vegetable Compound. There are also plant products that are intended to suppress menstruation itself. Their use is based on untested, anecdotal support. Black Cohosh goes by many names including black snakeroot and bugbane. Commonly used to treat "female disorders," it was one of the main constituents of Lydia Pinkham's Vegetable Compound and is also sold in many countries under the name "Remifemin." Extracts of Black Cohosh can bind to estrogen receptors in the pituitary gland and can suppress LH, the ovulation hormone, but there are no studies to support claims of its effectiveness in treating menstrual (or menopausal) symptoms.

Chinese traditional medicine has many plant products for female complaints. Dong Quai is the most commonly prescribed Chinese herbal medicine for this purpose. It is supposed to regulate and balance the menstrual cycle and strengthen the uterus. Another herbal product widely used for premenstrual syndrome is Evening Primrose, used either as the seeds of the plant or the expensive oil extract. A recent analysis of the available clinical trials of Evening Primrose oil for the treatment of premenstrual syndrome (PMS) found that all but one of the trials were inadequate for valid interpretation of the results. The one random-assignment, double-blind study available concluded that the active ingredient of Evening Primrose, gamma-linolenic acid, was ineffective in mitigating the symptoms of PMS.

There are many herbal products thought to have hormone-like activity, recommended for a range of reproduction-related problems including menstrual disorders, vaginal dryness, to reduce libido, increase libido, prolong lactation, induce abortion, prevent threatened abortion, or to control hot flushes and other vasomotor symptoms of the menopause. Though most of the therapeutics are ineffective or unproven, some may hold promise if tested properly. Meanwhile, there is no product from the realm of plant medicines that can be reliably used to suppress menstruation in order to eliminate menstrual cycle–related medical problems.

8

∞

In Support of Menstruation

Despite the documented disadvantages of regular menstrual cycles for the health and well-being of women, it is surprising that most of the books and articles on the subject, written by both women and men, have not recommended measures to suppress menstruation. Instead, it is the conformist attitude advocating the status quo that predominates. In the centuries-old tradition of Hippocrates and Galen, most modern scholars seem to adopt the view that since it is "natural" for women to menstruate, it must be good for their health. They seem to believe that "you can't fool Mother Nature!" The logic is that things natural, such as pain, physical or mental impairment, or even disease, should be accepted simply because they are natural. This attitude about menstruation prevails until today, at the end of the twentieth century. Instead of recognizing the uselessness of periodic bleeding, some doctors and scientists still seek to attribute advantages that it might bring to women's health. They conclude, for example, that menstruation accounts for the lower rates of certain disease conditions found in women compared to men. An argument frequently raised in support of this view is the recognized fact that women, during the reproductive years when they have menstrual cycles, have a lower risk than men of developing cardiovascular diseases and suffering heart attacks. It is only when women reach menopause and stop menstruating that they become as susceptible as men to these diseases. The observation is correct but the conclusion is wrong. What actually protects women from the cardiovascular diseases that affect men, particularly arteriosclerosis and heart attacks, is not repeated menstrual bleeding but estrogen, whose production by the ovaries virtually comes to an end at menopause. Women who take estrogen during menopause continue to protect their cardiovascular system against these diseases, even without menstruating.

The protection afforded by estrogen is brought about through several mechanisms, principally its capacity to maintain elevated levels of the high-density lipoproteins (HDL), which remove cholesterol from cells, preventing it from being deposited in the arteries and thus avoiding the formation of plaques or atheromas. In addition, the female hormones, with or without progesterone, reduce the risk of blood clots. This is because estrogens increase fibrinolysis and the production of coagulation inhibitors.

Another theory to explain the protective effect of menstruation for heart disease has been proposed by Dr. J. Sullivan, a Veterans Administration pathologist. He postulates a correlation between cardiovascular disease and iron stores in the body. According to Sullivan, regularly menstruating women have a very small iron reserve of only ten to forty micrograms of the iron-carrying protein, ferritin, per liter of blood. When they stop menstruating, this reserve increases two- or three-fold. On the other hand, men of forty-five years of age have reserves that women attain only when they reach seventy. At this age, women have just as much risk of heart attacks as men of fifty-five. Sullivan calculated that a woman loses five hundred milligram of ferritin-associated iron per year through menstruation, a quantity of iron that corresponds to the amount lost by a donor giving one pint of blood twice a year. He concluded that, if menstruation protects women from heart attacks, men and menopausal women who donate blood are equally protected.

With this reasoning, Sullivan created a new rationalization for the ancient belief that bleeding saves lives. His theory was first published in *The Lancet* in 1981 and again in the *American Heart Journal* in 1989, but did not enlist many converts. During the past fifteen years, epidemiological studies involving thousands of women in the United States and in Europe have confirmed what was already known in 1981. Dietary fats and cholesterol are the principal risk factors for the increase in cardiovascular disease in women, as they are in men.

Dr. Sullivan was not the first and will certainly not be the last to propose a health-based explanation to assure women that they should be pleased to menstruate, rather than recognize that it is unnecessary and useless blood loss. Another modern-day argument to justify blood loss, through menstruation or bloodletting, was based on the presumed benefit resulting from the fact that anemia creates adverse conditions for infectious agents, since these invading organisms require iron to develop. It has even been argued that malnutrition increases the body's resistance to infection. In an 1868 volume entitled *Lectures in Clinical Medicine*, a French doctor, A. Trousseau, declared that treating anemia could result in the patient's death, justifying his conclusion by citing cases among his own patients who had died after being treated for anemia with ferrous salts.

In the mid-twentieth century, a London symposium heard reports of the purported benefits of anemia in women because it was discovered that in some populations of pulmonary tuberculosis patients, there were more deaths among males than among females. The symposium report cited that in England in 1950, there were nearly ten thousand deaths among men suffering from tuberculosis and only about six thousand deaths among women. In other countries, particularly in the United States, the risk of dying from tuberculosis also seemed greater for men. However, this sex difference was not observed in all countries. In Holland, for example, where anemia among women was just as prevalent as among English and American women, there was no difference between the sexes in the death rate from tuberculosis. There are even reports from several countries of greater female mortality.

Harmful effects on health from an excess of iron in the body as a consequence of iron injections has also been used as an argument in defense of menstruation, just as it was used to justify ancient bloodletting. In fact, the author of a 1979 scientific publication proposing this idea entitled his article, "In Defense of Ancient Bloodletting." In 1970, Dr. H. McFarlane of the University of Manchester in England, reported that intramuscular injections of iron, given to under-nourished children to treat anemia, resulted in fatal infections. Reports from several African countries also revealed that iron injections caused an exacerbation of malaria. The explanation proposed for the phenomenon is that the excess of iron caused by the injections stimulates bacterial growth, since bacteria requires iron as does the anemic, infected individual. Under normal conditions, the body uses various defense mechanisms to remove serum iron from bacterial reach. When specialized leukocytes disintegrate after entrapping and destroying bacteria, they release a substance called interleukin-1. This stimulates the synthesis of ferritin, the protein that stores iron, taking it out of reach of the bacteria. The leukocytes also release lactoferrin, which rapidly sequesters free iron, making it unavailable for the metabolic processes involved in bacterial growth and reproduction. When there is an excess of iron administered intramuscularly, these mechanisms of defense become inadequate to remove the iron from the blood, it becomes available to bacteria, and they are able to proliferate rapidly.

What these observations show is that the use of iron injections for the treatment of anemia should be avoided. The body has its own mechanisms to ensure that the levels of iron are never greater than necessary. This obvious conclusion does not justify the defense of menstruation and its resultant anemia as a means for the body to defend itself against the deleterious effects of iron injections. There is no doubt, however, that an excess of iron in the blood, hyperferremia, can aggravate certain conditions. Professor E.

Weinberg, a microbiologist at the University of Indiana, has emphasized the toxic action of excess iron, particularly in sufferers of hemochromatosis and other conditions in which the mechanism of iron storage is impaired, leading to health problems for women. Among these conditions, Weinberg includes an excess of ingested iron, an increase in intestinal absorption caused by excessive alcohol or vitamin C consumption, parenteral iron administration (injections), and a reduction in the excretion of iron in premenopausal women following hysterectomy or during oral contraceptive pill use. Inclusion of hysterectomized women and of oral contraceptive pill users in this list is based on a weak argument. Quoting other authors (including the above-mentioned Sullivan), Weinberg alleges that the risk of cardiovascular disease increases for menopausal women and that when they undergo hysterectomy in the premenopause, this risk also increases in the last years before the menopause. Since hysterectomy is frequently accompanied by bilateral ovariectomy, the increased risk he describes could well be accounted for by the concomitant estrogen depletion. With respect to oral contraceptive users, the increase in risk of cardiovascular disease is unsubstantiated.

Articles describing menstrual bleeding as being good for women's health have appeared in magazines and newspapers, frequently written by women with premenstrual tension who experience relief from these symptoms with the arrival of their menstrual flow. Their conclusion is understandable; it is the conclusion of Hippocrates, echoing across the millennia.

Many gynecologists see menstruation as a protection against endometrial cancer or as a mechanism of eliminating an excess of iron or of toxins generated in women's bodies or derived from food. None of these ideas, however, are backed by actual facts. It is sometimes contended that the periodic shedding of the uterine lining is necessary to get rid of small nests of mutated cells that may lead to the growth of endometrial cancer. This idea does not take into account the fact that what is shed during menstruation is the outer layer of the endometrium, referred to as the functional layer. Endometrial cancer cells originate in the inner, or basal layer, which is not shed during menstruation. What protects the endometrium from cancer is progesterone and not menstrual bleeding.

An interesting and elaborate justification for menstruation has been proposed by Dr. M. Profet in a 1993 article published in the *Quarterly Review of Biology*. Profet's explanation is that menstruation represents a defense against microbes transported into the woman's body by spermatozoa. In her well-referenced article, the author recognizes that the supposition that menstruation represents the body's way of ridding itself of some ill-defined "contamination or pollution," is based more on superstition than science. She proposes, instead, that the merit of periodic menstruation is the antiseptic value of menstrual blood, which helps women defend against infection. Profet's publication has had wide media exposure. Journals and magazines all over the world carried discussions of her work. It seemed to offer some valid explanation for the purpose of repeated menstrual bleeding, but there are some weaknesses in her argument. Most difficult to explain in the context of her theory is the fact that throughout history and even today in less-industrialized cultures, women menstruate relatively rarely. This has been pointed out by the anthropologist Beverly Strassman, a major figure in the study of menstruation and one of the first scientists to recognize the connection between high number of menstrual cycles and adverse health effects.

Profet alleges that menstruation is a general phenomenon in nature and, if it is not perceived in all species of mammals, this is because bleeding is occult in the majority of them. Among the animals that Profet believes to menstruate but which have never been seen menstruating, are elephants, zebras, cows, and mares. Over the years, studies by expert anatomists, using both the conventional microscope and the electron microscope, fail to reveal evidence of menstrual-like bleeding in these species with different reproductive patterns than that of women. The comparative anatomy of the uterus is a well-studied subject that has attracted outstanding scientists such as Harvard Professor G. Wislocki, Professor E. Amoroso, from the West Indies, and Professor M. Burgos, from Argentina. Their work does not substantiate the idea of occult uterine bleeding in non-menstruating species. There is no relationship between menstruation and the so-called bleeding phase associated with the rupture of the ovarian follicle and "heat" of certain non-primate species such as the dog.

Profet concludes, "menstruation was planned to occur at the appropriate time to deal with the pathogens brought by the sperm. Menstruation follows sexual activity." Successful sexual activity in humans occurs in the peri-ovulatory period, from the tenth to the fourteenth day of the cycle. To wait from fifteen to twenty days to initiate an attack on pathogens in the female reproductive tract would be far too late. It is also relevant that we have no evidence that women who spend long periods of time in amenorrhea and are sexually active are more prone to infections.

Users of the contraceptive pill who have menstrual suppression have reduced risk of pelvic and vaginal infection. This observation makes it difficult to accept the thesis proposed by Profet. Contrary to her conclusion, menstrual blood is an excellent culture medium, permitting the development of toxic shock syndrome in users of tampons, which can lead to the user's death. Toxic shock syndrome is almost always caused by the production of one or more toxins at the site of a usually asymptomatic *Staphylococcus aureus* infection. The vagina is the most common site of the infection. The disease manifests itself during menstruation in users of vaginal tampons and the clinical picture is devastating. The patient suffers an extremely high fever, followed by muscular pain, nausea, vomiting, and uncontrollable diarrhea. During the first days, an extensive rash appears and the conjunctiva of the eyes become filled with blood. The general state of the patient deteriorates rapidly and when she reaches a doctor she is frequently in shock. In the 1980s, when the syndrome first appeared in association with super-absorbent tampons, around 10 percent of victims died. From then on, there were no further deaths thanks to better knowledge of the causes of shock, more rapid and efficient therapeutic measures, and the removal from the market of super-absorbent tampons.

A thoughtful analysis of sex differences in disease mortality was published in a 1998 issue of *Perspectives in Biology and Medicine*. The authors, Dr. Michel Garenne and Dr. Monique Lafon of Paris explain that in human populations females usually have a lower mortality than males at any age. This, incidentally, is true even before birth when there is a higher incidence of male fetal deaths than females in cases of miscarriage or spontaneous abortion. However, lower female mortality is not universal and a reverse pattern of excess female mortality has been observed for some infectious diseases, including tuberculosis, measles, whooping cough, diphtheria, and congenital syphilis. For many diseases, late childhood and early adulthood appear to be the life periods when females are the most vulnerable compared to males. The French scientists ascribe the difference in vulnerability to well-known differences between the male and female immune system, under the influence of the regulation of the sex hormones. Menstruation, per se, plays no role in either reducing or increasing the risk of infection.

One of the most imaginative suggestions to explain why women menstruate is that it provides women with vicarious sexual satisfaction, thus enabling them to preserve their virginity. The same author of that astounding proposition added the somewhat paradoxical view that another purpose was to get rid of unimplanted embryos. In recent years, a paper read at the American Anthropological Society suggested that the observation of the menstrual flow is used to confirm a woman's sexual potency.

Ultimately, the attitudes in support of menstruation come down not to medical reasons but to psychological and sociological factors, passed down through the centuries. It is associated with a girl "coming of age," entering the phase of femininity and fertility. An interesting case out of Eastern culture comes from Nepal where a child Goddess is ordained at age four, selected because she is believed to possess a divine spirit. She is worshiped by the nation until she begins to menstruate, a sign that her godly power is departing as she becomes a woman.

Absence of Menstruation and Disease

The absence of menstruation in women of reproductive age is considered a sign of disease and should be treated as an abnormality if the woman is neither pregnant nor breast-feeding. Menstruation will not occur, for example, in the case of congenital absence of the uterus, an anomaly that occurs in one in five thousand women. This defect is generally noticed when a woman reaches sixteen or seventeen years of age without menstruating. Resulting from a defect in fetal development of the reproductive system, absence of the uterus is generally accompanied by absence of the vagina. Since the ovaries function normally, ovulating and cyclically producing hormones, these women are otherwise normal in all respects. Surgical intervention to create an artificial vagina resolves the sexual problem. Assisted reproduction procedures now make it possible for these women to have children, using their own eggs and a surrogate mother's uterus to gestate the externally inseminated egg.

Other defects of the uterus can result in a lack of menstruation. Very small uteri have an insufficiently developed endometrium. Because of the absence of essential hormone receptors, this type of hypoplastic or infantile uterus does not respond adequately to the stimulating action of sexual hormones. Another condition is the syndrome of testicular feminization, a genetic abnormality causing the absence of uterus, vagina, fallopian tubes, and ovaries. In fact, the individual with this genetic abnormality has undescended testes either in the abdominal cavity or the inguinal canal. At birth the infant is believed to be a female and is raised as a girl. Usually seen by a doctor as young women, patients with this syndrome are actually genetically male, with testicles that produce the male hormone, testosterone. However, the organs that should be masculinized by the action of this hormone do not respond because they do not have specific androgen receptors due to a genetic defect. The male hormone is transformed into the female hormone, which, in turn, transforms the genetic male into an individual with the characteristics of a woman. In these cases, the abdominal testicles should be removed because of the high risk of malignant tumors, and supplementation of female hormones should be given so that the individual can continue to live as a woman. Surgical creation of an artificial vagina can be achieved successfully.

Enzymatic deficiencies can also interfere with the synthesis of the female hormone, causing absence of uterus, vagina, and breasts. One of the most serious deficiencies results in the inability of either the ovaries or adrenal glands to synthesize sex hormones. Carriers of this genetic defect have neither uterus nor breasts and the ovaries appear to be abdominal testicles that do not produce testosterone. The woman's appearance is distinctly female despite the absence of breasts.

When menstruation never begins, amenorrhea is referred to as primary. In so-called secondary amenorrhea, absence of menstruation is noticed after menstrual periods have started. Traumatic amenorrhea is one type of secondary amenorrhea. One frequent cause is overly aggressive curettage carried out to stop excessive uterine bleeding or to complete an incomplete abortion, or, in other cases, to induce an abortion. In some cases, the lesions caused by the procedure are transformed into scars that can reduce the endometrial surface, leaving insufficient lining tissue to create a menstrual flow. The condition is named the Asherman syndrome after the British doctor who described a great number of cases. Scarring close to the lower part of the uterus can cause obstruction of the cervix, thus preventing menstruation even when there is still sufficient endometrium. In these cases, menstrual blood accumulates in the uterus, drains through the fallopian tubes into the abdominal cavity, and is re-absorbed without the woman being aware of it. It is also possible for blood to remain in the uterus and to accumulate in the vagina when the hymen has no opening (imperforated hymen).

In addition to the congenital absence of a uterus or traumatic scarring of the uterus resulting in amenorrhea, there are various ovarian abnormalities that can cause primary or secondary amenorrhea. Defects in ovarian development are responsible for more than half the cases of primary amenorrhea. Viral infections such as mumps can cause ovarian lesions leading to secondary amenorrhea and premature menopause.

Ovarian Dysfunction

The most frequent error in ovarian development is Turner's syndrome, first described in 1938. It is a genetically induced developmental abnormality that generally results in sexual infantilism, low stature, and amenorrhea. The gonads do not develop and the germ cells, which normally would give rise to the ovary's eggs, degenerate (undergo atresia) during fetal life. The gonads appear as streaks of white tissue situated adjacent to the fallopian tubes. They do not produce hormones. There are many physical variations of Turner's syndrome. The characteristics most common to the syndrome are shortness of height, amenorrhea, and sparse sexual development. In addition, the patient's neck is wider at its base, similar to the silhouette of the Sphinx of Egypt, and the patient's chest is shield-shaped. Defects in the cardiovascular system are frequently seen in these patients. These women have a chromosomal constitution of 45,X which means they suffer from a deletion of chromosomal material from the X chromosomes. Gonadal tumors are rare in these cases so that it is not necessary to remove the non-functional streak gonads. There is another variant, which has a genetic mosaicism that includes Y chromosomal material and normal 46,XX cells. They may not have all the typical symptoms of Turner's syndrome but they do have classical gonadal dysgenesis. When genetic analysis reveals this situation, the streak gonads should be removed because they have a high incidence of gonadal tumors originating in these non-functional organs.

Premature Menopause

Premature ovarian failure is another cause of amenorrhea. This is responsible for 10 percent of cases of secondary amenorrhea and, because of its generally irreversible nature, it is considered early or premature menopause when it occurs in patients under forty years of age. Premature termination of ovarian activity is generally accompanied by all the symptoms of menopause (hot flushes, night sweats, vaginal dryness, depression), and can lead to osteoporosis, an increased risk of cardiovascular disease, and the much-feared Alzheimer's disease. Patients with premature menopause are generally women who began menstruating late and who menstruated irregularly. Ovarian dysfunction frequently occurs with the simultaneous dysfunction of other glands, principally the thyroid and adrenal glands. In other cases, the dysfunction can be associated with infection or surgery. Lesions that damage vasculature or ovarian innervation can result in ovarian failure. Autoimmune mechanisms which destroy the receptors of the pituitary hormones that make the ovaries work, can also explain some cases of premature menopause.

Treatment of premature ovarian failure consists basically in replacing the ovarian hormones. Menopausal symptoms, as well as the risk of osteoporosis and of the other risks linked to the menopause, disappear with hormone replacement therapy. Even periodic bleeding episodes similar to menstruation can be provoked with the suspension of hor-

mone administration to satisfy the psychological requirements of some women who associate bleeding with femininity. Most women, however, opt for hormone replacement
therapy without bleeding.

Pituitary Gland Dysfunction

Since the ovaries depend on the stimulus of the pituitary
hormones (FSH and LH) to function, it is obvious that pituitary abnormalities that alter the production or the secretion of these gonadotropic hormones interfere with ovarian
function. Deficiencies in gonadotropin production can occur
for various reasons, the most frequent being vascular lesions
or tumors. Sheehan's syndrome, for example, is a deficiency
in the production of gonadotropins resulting from pituitary
necrosis which develops in some women who suffer hemorrhage and shock during or after labor. These women are
unable to breast-feed because the necrotic pituitary does not
produce prolactin and oxytocin, hormones which are required for lactation. Subsequently, most patients with Sheehan's syndrome no longer ovulate or menstruate.

The degree of damage to the pituitary in patients with
Sheehan's syndrome will define the extent of ovarian deficiency. In extreme cases, there is also loss of thyroid and
adrenal function because these two glands, just as the ovary,
are controlled by protein hormones sent through the bloodstream by the pituitary.

Other conditions that can result in pituitary failure and
ovarian inactivity are a result of a massive swelling of the
gland because of hemorrhage or a tumor, and the so-called
empty sella syndrome, which is the result of a structural
defect in the concavity, the sella turcica, where the pituitary
is situated. When this defect occurs, the sella can fill up with
cerebrospinal fluid, which can give a radiological impression
that the sella is empty. In the enlarged sella–empty sella
syndrome, the pituitary tissue is actually flattened in the
floor of the sella, maintaining some part of its normal

hormone production so that the women may or may not have endocrine abnormalities. This syndrome is more common in obese women who usually have high blood pressure and complain of headaches. It can also occur following surgery or radiation.

Primary pituitary tumors that can reduce the production of gonadotropins include gliomas, craniopharyngiomas, meningiomas, as well as metastases of tumors in other parts of the body. Some tumors secrete increased quantities of gonadotropic hormones. In these cases, there is also an interruption in ovarian cyclic activity and consequently amenorrhea occurs. The most common of all these tumors are prolactin-producing adenomas, called prolactinomas. Elevated levels of prolactin inhibit both gonadotropin-releasing hormone (LHRH) and the secretion of FSH and LH. The low levels of gonadotropins, and consequently of estrogen, make ovulation and menstruation impossible. Amenorrhea generally occurs together with an abundant secretion of milk from the mammary glands, giving rise to the name galactorrhea-amenorrhea syndrome.

Most benign prolactinomas are very small and are referred to as microprolactinomas. Except for amenorrhea and galactorrhea associated with anovulation and consequently with infertility and a lower libido, bearers of microprolactinomas have no other symptoms. However, when the tumors are large, macroprolactinomas, other symptoms emerge, resulting from the compression and dislocation of neighboring tissues such as optic nerves. The patient may suffer headaches as well as reduction of the visual field. Other causes of hypersecretion of prolactin should be investigated whenever the syndrome of galactorrhea-amenorrhea is diagnosed. Among them, the most important are hypothyroidism, pregnancy, and the use of tranquilizers and anti-depressives. Prolactinomas regress under the action of dopamine agonists such as bromocriptine, an ergot derivative which can be administered by either oral or vaginal route.

Another type of hormone-secreting tumor, the ACTH-secreting adenoma overstimulates the adrenal gland, causing an excess of cortisone-like hormones. This inhibits ovulation and consequently menstruation. Women with this kind of tumor generally have an appearance similar to patients with Cushing's syndrome: obesity, hirsutism, stretch marks on their body, and a "full-moon" face. The most efficient treatment is surgical removal of the tumor. After surgery, some patients still do not ovulate or menstruate because they develop polycystic ovaries during their illness and this also requires specific treatment.

Thyroid-stimulating-hormone (TSH) producing tumors also can cause anovulation and amenorrhea. The inhibiting effect is caused by an increase in prolactin causing the galactorrhea-amenorrhea syndrome, just as happens with prolactinomas. However, in this case, there is also hypothyroidism, which permits rapid diagnosis. TSH-producing tumors, just as prolactinomas, respond well to bromocriptine.

Hypothalamic Dysfunction

The hypothalamus is the floor of the midbrain where the small peptide hormones controlling the pituitary gland are produced and/or stored. Pituitary defects can be the result of hypothalamic dysfunction. This condition is regarded as secondary pituitary dysfunction. The hypothalamic peptide hormone which stimulates gonadotropin secretion (FSH and LH) is called LHRH (luteinizing-hormone-releasing-hormone) or GnRH (gonadotropin-releasing-hormone). The existence of a hypothalamic factor controlling the release of gonadotropic hormones was first discovered through brilliant experiments in ferrets carried out by the Oxford anatomist Geoffrey Harris in the 1940s. This started a feverish search for the structure of the factor, led by Roger Guillemin of the Salk Institute in La Jolla and Andrew Schally of New Orleans. Ultimately, the two shared the 1976 Nobel

Prize for Medicine for describing the ten amino acid structural formula of LHRH. The fascinating story of the twenty-year search for the structure of LHRH is told in the book *The Nobel Duel*, published in 1981.

Before Geoffrey Harris' work, anatomists believed that blood flowed from the pituitary gland's sella turcica, upward toward the hypothalamus. He showed that the opposite is the case and that hormones originating in the hypothalamus reach the pituitary through a microcirculatory portal system. It is not practical to tap this source to measure GnRH production levels. In human beings, the level of GnRH secretion can be measured indirectly by taking frequent measurements of LH levels in the peripheral blood. The diagnosis of GnRH dysfunction is generally made by eliminating the possibility of primary pituitary disease.

The kind of hypothalamic amenorrhea that has been most intensely studied is the type associated with a loss of body weight as a result of dietary restrictions, such as occurs in the disease of anorexia nervosa. This disorder occurs predominantly in Caucasian women under twenty-five years of age but less frequently affects men and women over age twenty-five. It is characterized by behavioral changes, extreme loss of weight, and amenorrhea. One in every hundred adolescents from affluent families develops this syndrome but women from any social group can be affected. The rate is especially high in ballet dancers who, as well as carrying out regular, intense physical exercise, are obliged to maintain a low body weight. The rate rises to 10 percent in all dancers and in the most competitive ballerinas it can rise to 20 percent. The most frequent symptoms of anorexia nervosa, in addition to extreme weight loss and amenorrhea, are low blood pressure, which occurs in 80 percent of patients, lower body temperature, observed in 65 percent, constipation, and dry hair and skin, found in more than 50 percent. Amenorrhea can begin as soon as dietary restrictions are imposed, even before a substantial weight loss occurs. In the majority, behavioral changes, including exaggerated preoccupation with weight and physical appearance, amenorrhea and weight loss occur simultaneously. Anorexia nervosa can occur together with bulimia or without it. Bulimia sufferers binge frequently on food (often eating great quantities in one sitting), then try to rid themselves of the food they have ingested by provoking vomiting or by using laxatives or diuretics.

Hormonally, a reduction in estrogen levels is observed in non-bulimic patients as a result of ovarian inactivity. This is a consequence of low levels of the pituitary gonadotropins, FSH and LH, reflecting the absence of the pulsatile secretion of GnRH. The administration of a pulsatile infusion of this hormone can re-initiate ovulation and consequently menstruation. However, the correct treatment of a patient with anorexia nervosa requires nutritional and psychotherapeutical support, fostering a change of attitude toward the body.

Weight Loss

Simple weight loss caused by degenerative or infectious diseases or even of a nervous origin can cause inhibition of the pulsatile secretion of GnRH, resulting either in amenorrhea or in the occasional interruption of menstruation. Similarly, special diets can cause amenorrhea even when there is no restriction of calories and the diet consists only in qualitative changes and composition of food intake. Strict vegetarian diets, for example, are associated with high rates of menstrual irregularities and amenorrhea.

Genetic Defects

There are two syndromes associated with genetic defects which involve the hypothalamus and which result in primary amenorrhea: Kallman's syndrome (hypogonadotropic hypogonadism) is associated with lack of sense of smell (anosmia) and, in some cases, deafness. Lawrence-Moon-Biedl's syndrome is characterized by obesity, low stature, diabetes insipidus, mental retardation, and polydactylism. There are also non-hereditary syndromes that affect or involve hypothalamic alterations and can result in amenorrhea.

Although not experienced by most women, a relatively long period of anovulation and consequently of amenorrhea can occur following the suspension of hormonal contraceptive use or following abortion. The phenomenon is more common in women of low body weight who menstruate irregularly and is simply called post-pill amenorrhea when it occurs after stopping the use of the contraceptive pill, or post-abortion amenorrhea, when it occurs after the interruption of a pregnancy. It is also observed in women who discontinue the use of long-acting injectables such as DepoProvera®.

Polycystic Ovaries

Polycystic ovarian disease, also known as Stein-Leventhal's syndrome in recognition of the first scientists to describe seven cases of the disorder in 1935, is the disorder most frequently associated with long periods of amenorrhea, sometimes interrupted by bleeding episodes of long duration. Polycystic ovaries are present in around 20 to 25 percent of women. Multiple cystic follicles on the ovary's surface, however, is insufficient evidence to characterize the disease. It has the additional characteristics of menstrual disturbances caused by anovulation, particularly amenorrhea interspersed with periods of bleeding; obesity; a rise in the ovulation hormone, LH; a reduction in the follicular stimulating hormone, FSH; and androgynism, which is responsible for hirsutism (excessive growth of hair). Polycystic ovaries can also result in alterations in the function of the adrenal gland, characterized by an increase in the production of androgens (male sex hormones) because of a congenital deficiency of the enzymes responsible for the synthesis of corticosteroids. Late congenital adrenal hyperplasia is a condition that appears at adulthood, resulting also from a deficiency of several enzymes that are normally involved in corticosteroid production. By various hormone measurements, it is possible to distinguish between ovarian polycystic syndrome and congenital adrenal hyperplasia.

The treatment of polycystic ovaries aims principally at restoring the fertility of the patient. However, for many patients with this syndrome, the most important goal (which in reality should be the least important) is to restore menstruation. To achieve this, doctors create an artificial menstrual cycle by the intermittent use of oral contraceptive pills. The benefit of using contraceptive pills is actually based on their protective effect on the endometrium which, in the case of patients with polycystic ovaries who do not ovulate, is under hyperstimulation from the continuous action of high levels of ovarian estrogen. The continuous action of low-dose oral contraceptives would, therefore, assure the benefit without requiring the unnecessary inconvenience of menstruation.

For some women the most disturbing consequence of polycystic ovarian syndrome is hirsutism and not the lack of menstruation. These patients seek medical help to get rid of the excess hair. In these cases, treatment usually involves the administration of anti-androgen.

A more rational solution for treating patients with polycystic ovarian syndrome is to induce ovulation with clomiphene citrate, as proposed by Dr. Robert Greenblatt of Augusta, Georgia in 1961, and which has been widely used for the past forty years. This was actually a serendipitous finding. Greenblatt was testing in women the possible use of chlomiphene citrate as a contraceptive, following reports of laboratory results with experimental animals. To his surprise, among his volunteer patients, some with a history of anovulation responded to the drug by ovulating.

When drug treatment does not give satisfactory results, there still remains an option used first by one of the doctors whose name is associated with the syndrome, Dr. F. Stein.

He undertook a surgical reduction in the size of the polycystic ovaries by the removal of a slice of each ovary. The operation, sometimes referred to as a wedge resection of the ovary, is seldom used today.

In all the conditions described, the failure to menstruate is a symptom and not the underlying cause of the disease process. Treatment to artificially restore a simulated pattern of menstrual flow does nothing to resolve the underlying disease or the main problem, which usually is infertility. In fact, maintenance of amenorrhea until it is possible to restore ovulation can be beneficial in some cases.

10

∽

Conclusion

Recurrent menstruation is unnecessary and can be harmful to the health of women. It is a needless loss of blood.

Menstruation is responsible for aggravating an array of menstrual cycle–related medical disorders and is the cause of serious diseases such as premenstrual syndrome and endometriosis. Menstruation exacerbates anemia, which afflicts millions of women around the world. Long menstruation-free periods, such as occur during pregnancy and breast-feeding, alleviate menstrual cycle–related diseases. Freeing women of menstruation significantly reduces the risk of life-threatening disease such as ovarian and uterine (endometrial) cancers. The longer a woman is not menstruating, the greater the benefit. Freedom from menstruation can be achieved by the use of long-acting contraceptives or continuous use of the oral contraceptive pill. Under proper medical supervision, it can also be attained through natural means such as a conscientious regimen of rigorous physical exercise.

Except for anemia, which has been known since the time of Hippocrates, the most debilitating consequences of repeated menstruation were recognized only in the twentieth century. Premenstrual tension undoubtedly existed in the past, but its association with menstruation itself was not recognized. Women with PMS were often considered witches or mentally disturbed. Some of these unfortunate women were confined to insane asylums or even sentenced to be burned at the stake.

The relationship between menstruation and endometriosis was first described in 1927, while associations between menstruation and other catamenial diseases were recognized even more recently. Meanwhile, menstrual cycle–related medical diseases are now appearing more frequently because modern women are menstruating more often than women did in the past. Today's woman has her first menstrual period earlier in life, has fewer children, and has them at a later age. Moreover, diagnostic tools such as ultrasonography, laparoscopy, and hysteroscopy permit earlier detection of these diseases. Menstrual cycle–related problems account for fully 50 percent of women's gynecological complaints. Currently, some women must have their menstruation suppressed because of extreme pain, excessive blood loss, migraine, or other symptoms associated with menstrual cycle–related illness. There are many other women who may consider menstruation suppression as a way to prevent the development of these conditions.

Anemia remains one of the most serious health problems in the world. A study published in the *Journal of the American Medical Association (JAMA)* reports that 9 percent of all toddlers and about 10 percent of adolescent girls of childbearing age in the United States are iron-deficient. These prevalence rates correspond to over seven and a half million girls and young women with iron deficiency. By contrast, this deficiency is present in no more than 1 percent of teenage boys and young men. The authors point out that after the recognition of this epidemic of iron deficiency in the United States in the late 1960s efforts were intensified toward its prevention. However, iron deficiency still remained prevalent in women of childbearing age in the late '70s when iron deficiency was last assessed nationally. This *JAMA* publication confirms that iron deficiency is a problem mainly for menstruating women and their very young children.

The problem of anemia in less affluent countries of eastern and southern Europe and in many other developing countries remains much worse. Considering that the monthly loss of blood is absolutely needless and that the treatment of anemia significantly increases the cost of the already overburdened health services of these countries, the suppression of menstruation would be an important public health measure, as well as a health benefit to individual women.

We envisage a campaign involving both the public and private sectors, engaging the medical profession to educate the public about the uselessness of menstruation for women not actively seeking pregnancy. The campaign could be promoted in parallel with family-planning programs that inform women of the benefits of oral hormonal contraceptives and long-acting products that inhibit ovulation. The choices include injectable progestins, subdermal implants, and progestin-releasing intrauterine systems.

Women are ahead of policy makers and industry executives in becoming receptive to these ideas. The International Health Foundation recently described the results of a survey of nearly one thousand five hundred women of reproductive age concerning the impact of commonly used contraceptive methods on mood, sex life, and menstruation as well as their satisfaction and concerns regarding birth control methods. The respondents were also asked about their reaction to hypothetical methods. Sixty-two percent of current oral contraceptive users expressed interest in a schedule of withdrawal bleeding every three months. Total suppression of bleeding was favored by almost one-half the respondents. Those preferring to continue the usual monthly schedule gave as reasons for that preference, "to allow the body to function normally," "to rid the body of wastes," and "to confirm that you are not pregnant." The reasons cited in favor of reducing the frequency of menstruation were that it was "an inconvenience" or "a hassle." None of the women surveyed mentioned the possible benefits to their health of the suppression of repeated bleeding. Nevertheless, almost half of them indicated their willingness to use a pill that would keep them free of menstruation.

Delaying the age of menarche can have both personal and social ramifications. Although precocious puberty is defined usually as puberty before the age of ten years, from a social point of view becoming a reproductively competent woman before fifteen years of age presents no advantage whatsoever for most girls in Western cultures. The postponement of menarche by delaying activation of the hormonal axis that triggers ovulation can add several menstruation-free years in a young girl's life when being sexually developed is neither necessary nor without risk.

In countries where the age of menarche is early, pregnancies in very young girls are common. Nearly one million U.S. teenagers become pregnant each year and about five hundred thousand give birth. Young girls aged ten to fourteen are part of this statistic. Each year about twelve thousand of these children have babies. Ongoing enthusiastic campaigns urging teens to delay sexual activity until they are older may have limited success, at best. The National Survey of Family Growth finds that the proportion of adolescent girls experiencing sexual intercourse declined from 53 percent to 50 percent between 1988 and 1995. At this rate of decline, adolescent pregnancy in the United States will continue to be a problem for a long time.

In Brazil, almost thirty thousand pregnancies in girls age ten and eleven were reported in 1995. Family members and friends impregnated most of these girls. A girl's biological father was often the sexual assailant. The direct solution to this problem, which should be applied forcefully and without compromise, is to control the offenders or to remove them from the home. The combination of sexual maturity and youthful vulnerability puts young pre-adolescents living under the same roof as sexual predators at great risk. A later menarche is no guarantee of protection, but if delays her pubertal changes, the young girl may be less likely to be targeted and victimized by sexual harassment and abuse. Many studies show that the menarche comes at an older age for girls who undertake a regular program of physical exercise starting around eight years of age and that this is not accompanied by other undesirable effects on health.

The proposition of menstruation suppression may be interpreted by some as contrary to a fundamental law of nature. The attitude that menstruation is a "natural event" and therefore beneficial to women in some way has no basis in scientific fact. Since antiquity, a woman became pregnant near the time of the menarche (which was quite late by today's standards) and remained menstruation-free for the rest of her short life, because of continuous cycles of pregnancy and lactation. Regular and recurrent menstruation throughout most of a woman's reproductive years is a fairly recent phenomenon. It has come about because of reduction in the length of time that women intensively nurse their babies and the steadily declining birth rate. This began in Europe and North America after the industrial revolution and more recently in the world's less developed regions. The indispensable feature of life is reproduction. Menstruation is an unnecessary, avoidable byproduct of the human reproductive process.

The transition to a new reproductive paradigm cannot be achieved overnight, but by the gradual transformation of the old. In this book we propose the abandonment of the traditional paradigm, ordained by Hippocrates in an era of medical naivete, that regular menstruation is good for women. Understanding why cyclical bleeding is unnecessary would be the next step. This would be followed by more women becoming comfortable with the idea of not menstruating. With the cooperation and supervision of their physicians, women would use currently available means to stop menstruation for several months and, growing more confident, would lengthen the menstruation-free interval. As the benefits become evident, other women would be encouraged to try this procedure and medical researchers would be motivated to find more advanced methods to control menstruation. This would forge a major advance in women's health, led by women. Today's proposal would become tomorrow's new paradigm. The pioneer feminist Margaret Sanger wrote, "No woman is completely free unless she has control over her own reproductive system."

Let this new freedom begin.

Glossary

ADENOMYOSIS   endometriosis affecting the uterine muscle

ADRENAL CORTICOTROPIC HORMONE (ACTH)   pituitary hormone that stimulates the adrenal gland to produce cortisone

AMENORRHEA OR AMENORRHEIC   not menstruating

ANDROGYNISM   mosaic of male and female characteristics

ANDROSTENEDIONE   precursor of the male hormone testosterone

ANEMIA   low iron levels in the blood

ANOREXIA NERVOSA   a severe eating disorder characterized by the fear of weight gain leading to faulty eating patterns, weight loss, and often anovulation

ANOSMIA   absence of sense of smell

ANOVULATION   failure to ovulate

ATRESIA   natural disintegration of egg cells within the ovary

BULIMIA   an eating disorder characterized by periods of binging (eating huge quantities) and purging (vomiting, using laxatives). It is frequently associated with disruption of the hormones of reproduction

CATAMENIAL   recurring monthly at the time of the menstruation

CHOLECYSTECTOMY   operation to remove the gall bladder

CORPUS LUTEUM   the vacated ovarian follicle that produces progesterone

CORTICOSTEROID   hormones (i.e. cortisone) produced by outer layer of adrenal gland

CORTISOL   steroid hormone produced by the adrenal gland

DECIDUA   the uterine lining cells just before menstruation

DIHYDROEPIANDROSTERONE (DHEA)   a precursor of androgens, the male sex hormones

DIMORPHISM   different bodily structure, such as height or muscle mass, between males and females

DYSMENORRHEA   menstrual cramps

DYSPAREUNIA   pain associated with coitus

EMESIS   vomiting

ENDOMETRIOMAS   nests of misplaced uterine cells that cause endometriosis

ENDOMETRIOSIS   a painful disease that occurs when uterine lining cells (endometrium) grow somewhere else in the body (usually on other pelvic organs)

ENDORPHINS   naturally produced substances that affect the brain similarly to opioids

ESTROGEN   the main female sex hormone produced by the ovary

FIBRINOGEN   a blood protein that participates in clot formation

FOLLICLE (OVARIAN)   the structure within the ovary that contains an egg

FOLLICLE-STIMULATING-HORMONE (FSH)   pituitary hormone that stimulates estrogen production by the ovary

GALACTORRHEA   abnormal milk production by mammary gland due to prolactin

GONADOTROPIN-RELEASING HORMONE (GnRH)   peptide hormone that causes the pituitary gonadotropins (LH and FSH) to be released. It is also called LHRH

HEMOCHROMATOSIS   a blood disease that leads to the accumulation of iron in tissues

HEMOSTASIS   stabilization of blood circulation

HUMAN CHORIONIC GONADOTROPIN (HCG)   the placental hormone of pregnancy

HYPOXIA   oxygen deprivation

HYSTERECTOMY   surgical removal of the uterus

INGUINAL CANAL   opening between the scrotum and floor of the pelvic cavity

LUTEINIZING HORMONE (LH)   pituitary hormone that stimulates the ovary and brings about ovulation

MEIOSIS   the specialized division of cells that will form sperm or eggs and reduce the chromosome number by half

MENARCHE   a woman's first menstruation, at puberty

MENOPAUSE   the end of menstruations because of the depletion of eggs in the ovary

MITOCHONDRIA   sub-cellular structure within the cytoplasm of every cell

MITOSIS   the process of cell division that results in two identical daughter cells

MYOMA   a benign fibroid tumor in the uterine muscle

MYOMETRIUM   muscle layer of the uterus

NEOPLASIA   a malignant tumor

OLIGOMENORRHEA   infrequent or irregular menstruations

OOPHORECTOMY   surgical removal of the ovaries

OVARIECTOMY   surgical removal of the ovaries

OXYTOCIN   a hormone produced by the pituitary gland that causes uterine contractions

PHAGOCYTOSIS   incorporation of foreign organisms by defending immune cells

PHLEBOTOMY   opening of a vein for bloodletting

PLACEBO   a dummy drug or procedure used in clinical trials

PLETHORA   in medical usage, an excess of blood

PLEURISY   accumulation of fluid in the lung

POLYCYSTIC OVARIES   abnormal condition involving lack of ovulation and infertility

PROGESTERONE   the steroid hormone necessary to maintain pregnancy

PROLACTIN   a pituitary hormone that induces lactation and prevents ovulation

PROSTAGLANDIN   hormone with many bodily effects including contracting smooth muscle

PULSATILE SECRETION   pattern of hormone secretion that creates bursts instead of a steady flow. It is characteristic of the way GnRH and some pituitary hormones are released

SELLA TURCICA   concavity at base of the midbrain where the pituitary gland is situated

SEROTONIN   a naturally produced substance that is involved in nerve signal transmission

STROMA   one of the cell types of the uterine lining

THALASSEMIA   genetic disease that causes destruction of red blood cells

THROMBOCYTOPENIA   a blood disorder that destroys platelets so that blood does not clot

THROMBOPHLEBITIS   blood clot in a vein of the leg

TRANSFERRIN   the blood protein that transfers iron from the circulation into hemoglobin

UTERINE ATROPHY   shrinkage of the uterus

VENESECTION   opening of a vein with the use of a scalpel or lancet

VENOUS THROMBOSIS   blood clot in any vein

Bibliographic Essay

Included in the endnotes are citations of key books and publications that are the basis for many of the facts and conclusions presented. Readers now have access to most of the medical literature through the Internet so we have included not only reference books available in most general libraries, but citations that can be found in original publications in medical journals. This database can be accessed at no cost, courtesy of the U.S. National Library of Medicine by entering http//www.ncbi.nlm.nih.gov/PubMed/ through most search engines.

INTRODUCTION

The evolution of human reproduction. Short, R. *Proceedings of the Royal Society of London* 195:3–25, 1976; Hippocratic writings. *Great Books of the Western World*. *No. 10*. McHutchins, R., editor-in-chief. Encyclopedia Britannica, Inc., 1952; *Blood Magic. The Anthropology of Menstruation*. Buckley, T., and Gottlieb A., eds. University of California Press, Los Angeles, 1988; *Galen on Bloodletting*. Brain, P. Cambridge University Press, Cambridge, 1986; In defense of ancient bloodletting. Brain, P. *S. Afr. Med. J.* 56:149–154, 1979; *Full Moons*. Katzeff, P. Citadel Press, Secaucus, NJ, 1981; *The Principles and Practice of Medicine*. Osler, W. The Classics of Medicine Library. Division of Gryphon Editions Ltd., Birmingham, AL, 1978; Reversible sterility induced by medroxyprogesterone injections. Coutinho, E. M., de Souza, J. C., and Csapo, A. I. *Fertil. Steril.* 17:261, 1966; A Comparative study of intermittent versus continuous use of a contraceptive pill administered by vaginal route. Coutinho, E. M, O'Dwyer, E., Barbosa, I. C, Gu, Z. P., and Shaaban, M. M. *Contraception* 51:355, 1995; Packaging the pill. Gossel, P. In *Encounter with Technology: Health, Medicine and the Artifact*. Bud, R., Finn, B., and Trischler, eds. Harwood Academic Publishers, 1997; *Patterns and Perceptions of Menstruation*. A World Health Organization international study. Snowden, R., and Christian, B., eds. St. Martin's Press, New York, 1983; Teenage Pregnancy in the United States. *The Guttmacher Report on Public Policy* 1:5, Alan Guttmacher Institute, New York, October 1998.

CHAPTER 1: MENSTRUATION IN WESTERN CIVILIZATION

Porneia: On Desire and the Body of Antiquity. Rousselle, A. Barnes & Noble Books, New York, 1996; *Histoire de la vie privée, vol. I. De L'Empire Romain à l'an mil.* Aries, P., and Duby, G. Editions du Seuil, Paris, 1985; *The Oldest Profession: A History of Prostitution.* Basser, L. Dorset Press, New York, 1993; *The Western Medical Tradition 800 BC to AD 1800.* Conrad, L. I., Neve, M., Nutton, V., Porter, R., and Wear, A. Cambridge University Press, Cambridge, 1995; *Sex in History.* Tannahill, R. Scarborough House Publishers, New York, 1992; *Quarderni d'Anatomia III. Organidella Generazione-Embrione.* da Vinci, L. Dodici Foglia della Royal Library di Windsor. Casa Editrice Jacob Dyburad. Christiana, 1513; *De Humani Corporis Fabrica.* Basilae, V. A. (facsimile Bruxelles, 1964), p. 1543; *William Harvey and the Circulation of Blood.* Whitteridge, G. MacDonald, London, and American Elsevier, New York, 1971; *An Anatomical Description of the Human Gravid Uterus and Its Contents.* Hunter, W. J. Johnson, London, 1794; Die innere Sekretion von ovarium und placenta. Halban, J. *Archiv für Gynaekologie* 75:353–441, 1905; Uber die Hormone Hypophysenvorderlapens. Zondek, B. *Klin. Wschr* 9:245–682, 1930; Physiology of the corpus luteum. II. Production of a special uterine reaction (progestational prolification) by extracts of the corpus luteum. Corner, G. W., and Allen, W. M. *Am. J. Physiol.* 88: 326, 1929; The human uterine mucous membrane during menstruation. Bartelmez, G. W. *Am. J. Obstet. Gynecol.* 21:623–643, 1931; Some problems related to ovarian function and to pregnancy. Zondek, B. *Recent Progress in Hormone Research*, Academic Press New York and London, 10:395–423, 1954.

CHAPTER 2: MENSTRUATION: THE BASIS OF THERAPEUTIC BLOODLETTING

Hippocrates. J. Jouanna, Fayard, Paris, 1992; *The Medical Works of Hippocrates.* Hippocrates. Blackwell, Oxford, 1950; Hippocrates and School of Cos. Between myth and skepticism. Joly, R. In *Nature Animated II.* Ruse, M., ed., Dordrecht, 1983; Sur l'origine hippocratique des concepts de revulsion e de derivation. Marganne, M. E. *L'Antiquite Classique* 49: 115–130, 1980; The female sex: Medical treatment and biological theories in the fifth and fourth centuries BC. *Science Folklore and Ideology, Part III.* Lloyd, G. Cambridge University Press, Cambridge, 1983; *Hippocratic Writings.* W. Benton, Publisher. Adams, F., trans. In *Great Books of the Western World*, Encyclopedia Britannica, Inc., Chicago, 1952; *Galen's System of Physiology and Medicine.* Siegel, R. E. Basel, 1968; *Galen on Bloodletting.* Brain, P. Cambridge University Press, 1986; In defense of ancient bloodletting. Brain, P. *S. Afr. Med. J.* 56:149–154, 1979; Anatomical disquisition on the motion of the heart and blood in animals. Harvey, W. 1628. In *Great Books of the Western World.* Hutchins, R. M., ed. No. 28. Encyclopedia Britannica, Inc., Chicago, 1952; The history of bloodletting. Kluger, M. J. *Natural History* 87:78–83, 1978; Erasistratus. Dobson, J. F. *Proc. Royal Soc. Med.* 3:825–832, 1927; Researches principally relative to the morbid and curative effects of loss of blood. Hall, M. 2nd American edition, Carey–Hart, Philadelphia, 1835; *The History of Obstetrics and Gynecology.* O'Dowd, M. J., and Philby, E. E., eds. Parthenon Publishing Group, London, 1994; *A Treatise on the Art of Cupping.* Mapleson, T., Cupper to His Majesty. John Wilson, London, 1830; *The Bloodletting Letter of 1539.* Bruxellensis, A. V. An annotated translation by John B. de C. M. Saunders and O'Malley, C. D. Henry Schuman, New York; *On the Proper Administration of Bloodletting for the Prevention and Cure of Disease.* Clutterbuck, H. S. Highley, London, 1840; *The Principles and Practice of Medicine.* Osler, W. Special edition printed privately for the *Classics of Medicine Library,* Division of Gryphon Editions Ltd., Birmingham, AL, 1978.

CHAPTER 3: WHY WOMEN MENSTRUATE
The emergence of modern humans. Stringer, C. B. *Sci. Am.* 263(6):98–104, 1990; Primate evolution: in and out of Africa. Stewart, C. B., and Disotell, T. R. *Current Biology* 8:582–588, 1998. The genetical archaeology of the human genome. von Haeseler, A. et al. *Nat. Genet.* 14(2): 135–40, 1996; Genetic traces of ancient demography. Harpending, H. C. et al. *Proc. Nat. Acad. Sci.* 95(4):1961–1967, 1998; Why do women and some other primates menstruate? Finn, C. A. *Perspect. Biol. Med.* 30:566–574, 1987; Menstruation: a non-adaptive consequence of uterine evolution. Finn, C. A. *Perspect. Biol. Med.* 73:163–173, 1998; *Mechanisms of Menstrual Bleeding.* Baird, D. T., and Michie, E. A., eds. Raven Press, New York, 1985; Physiology of the normal menstrual cycle. Barbieri, R. L. In *Modern Management of Premenstrual Syndrome.* Smith, S., and Schiff, I., eds., W. W. Norton & Co., New York, 1993; The ovarian triad of the primate menstrual cycle. Goodman, A. L., and Hodgen, G. D. *Recent Progress Hormone. Res.* 39:1–14, 1983; Hormonal relationships during the menstrual cycle. Yen, S. C. C., Vela, P., Rankin, J., et al. *JAMA* 211:1513–1519, 1970; *Coagulacao do sangue menstrual.* Salvatore, C. A. Livraria Roca, Sao Paulo, 1982; The fibrinolytic activity of the human endometrium. Albrechtsen, O. K. *Acta Endocrinolgica* 23:207–218, 1956; Retrograde menstruation in healthy women and in patients with endometriosis. Halme, J., Hammond, M. G., Hulka, J. F., Raj, S. J., and Talbert, L. M. *Obstet. Gynecol.* 64:151–154, 1984; Tubal and uterine motility. Coutinho, E. M. In *Nobel Symposium 15, 1971: Control of Human Fertility.* Diczfalusy, E., and Borell, U., eds. Almqvist and Wiksell, Stockholm, and John Wiley & Sons, New York.

CHAPTER 4: PREMENSTRUAL SYNDROME
The Menstrual Cycle. Dalton, K. First American edition. Pantheon Books, New York, 1969; *Once a Month.* Dalton, K. 2nd revised edition. Hunter House Inc. Publishers, Claremont, CA, 1988; *The Premenstrual*

Syndrome. Keye, Jr., W. R. W. B. Saunders Co., Philadelphia, 1988; *Premenstrual, Post-Partum and Menopausal Mood Disorders.* Demers, L. M., McGuire, J. L., Phillips, A., and Rubinow, D. R. Urban & Schwarzenberg, Baltimore, 1989; *Menstruation & Menopause.* Weideger, P. Alfred Knopf, New York, 1976; *The Menstrual Cycle.* Vollmann, R. F. W. B. Saunders Co., Philadelphia, 1977; *The Curse: A Cultural History of Menstruation.* Delaney, J. Lupton, M. J., and Toth, E., rev. ed. University of Illinois Press, Chicago, 1988; *Periods: From Menarche to Menopause.* Golub, S. Sage Publications, Inc., Newbury Park, CA, 1992; *Full Moons.* Katzeff, P. Citadel Press, Secaucus, NJ, 1981; *Premenstrual Syndrome and You.* Lauersen, N. H. and Stukane, E. Simon & Schuster, Inc., New York, 1983; The relationship of menstrually-related mood disorders to psychiatric disorders. Byrne, R., Hoban, P. P., and Rubinow, M. C., *Clin. Obstet. Gynecol.* 30:386–390, 1987; *The Lunar Effect: Biological Tides and Human Emotions.* Lieber, A. Anchor Press/Doubleday, New York, 1978; *The Psychiatric Implications of Menstruation.* Gold, J. H., ed. American Psychiatric Press, Inc. Washington, 1985; Differential behavioral effects of gonadal steroids in women with and in those without premenstrual syndrome. Schmidt, P., et al. *N. Engl. J. Med.* 338(4):209–216, 1998; *Menstrual Health in Women's Lives.* Dan, A. J. and Lewis, L. L. University of Illinois Press, Chicago, 1992; *Modern Management of Premenstrual Syndrome.* Smith, S., and Schiff, I. eds. Norton Medical Books, New York, 1993; Lasting response to ovariectomy in severe intractable premenstrual syndrome. Casson, P., Hahn P. M., Van Vogt, D. A., et al. *Am. J. Obstet. Gynecol.* 162:99–102, 1990; The premenstrual syndrome: effects of medical ovariectomy. Muse, K. N., Cetal, N. S., Futterman, L. A., et al. *N. Engl. J. Med.* 311:1345, 1984; The premenstrual syndrome—diagnosis and management. Smith, S., and Schiff, I. *Fertil. Steril.* 52:527–532, 1989; *Menstrual Cramps.* Lark, S. M. Westchester Publishing Co., Los Altos, CA, 1993; *The Premenstrual Syndromes.* Gise, L. H., ed. Churchill Livingstone, New York, 1988; *The Pre-menstrual Syndrome and Progesterone Therapy.* Dalton, K. Year Book Medical Publishers, Chicago, 1977; Psychotropic medications as treatment of dysphoric premenstrual syndrome. Goldenstein, S., and Halbreich, V. In *Modern Management of Premenstrual Syndrome.* S., Smith, and Schiff, I., eds. W. W. Norton & Co., New York, 1993; *The Woman in the Body.* Martin, E. Beacon Press, Boston, 1992. *Issues of Blood.* Laws, S. Macmillan, New York, 1982.

CHAPTER 5: MENSTRUAL CYCLE–RELATED DISORDERS
Menstrual Cramps. Lark, S. Westchester Publishing Co., Los Altos, CA, 1993; Migraine and reproductive hormones throughout the menstrual cycle. Epstein, M. T. *The Lancet* 534, 1975; The effect of oral contraceptives on migraine. Whitty, C. W. N., Hockaday, J. M., and Whitty, M. M.

The Lancet 856, 1966; Estrogen withdrawal migraine. Sommerville, B. W. *Neurology* 25:239, 1975; Aphasia, hemiparesis and hemianesthesia in migraine. Jeliffe, S. E. *NY State J. Med.* 83:33, 1906; Asthme et menstruation. Claude, F., and Allemany Vall, R. *Presse Med.* 38:755, 1938; Morbidity in asthma in relation to the menstrual cycle. Eliasson, O., Scherzer, H. H., and DeGraff, A. C. *J. Allergy Clin. Immunol.* 77:87, 1986; Menstrual cyclic thrombocytopenia. Tomer, A., Schreiber, A. D., McMillan, R., et al. *Br. J. Haematol* 71:519, 1989; Thrombotic thrombocytopenic purpura: a ten-year experience. Cuttner, J. *Blood* 56:302, 1980; Hormonal dependent thrombotic thrombocytopenic purpura (TTP). Holdrinet, R. S. G., de Pauw, B. E., and Haanan, C. *Scan. J. Hematol.* 30:250, 1983; Onset of manifestations of hepatic porphyria in relation to the influence of female sex hormones. Zimmerman, T. S., McMillin, J. M., and Watson, C. J. *Arch. Intern. Med.* 118:229, 1966; Alterations in heme biosynthesis during the human menstrual cycle: studies in normal subjects and patients with latent and active acute intermittent porphyria. McColl, K. E. L., Wallace, A. M., Moore, M. R., et al. *Clin. Sci.* 62:183, 1982; Oral contraceptive agents and the management of acute intermittent porphyria. Perlroth, M. G., Marner, H. S., and Tschudy, D. P. *JAMA* 194: 1037, 1965; Danazol administration to females with menses associated exacerbations of acute intermittent porphyria. Lamon, J. L., Frykholm, B. C., Herrera, W., et al. *J. Clin. Endocrinol. Metab.* 48:123, 1979; Menstrual cyclicity of finger joint size and grip strength in patients with rheumatoid arthritis. Rudge, S. R., Kawanko, I. C., and Drury, P. L. *Ann. Rheum. Dis.* 42:425, 1983; Three patterns of catamenial epilepsy. Herzog, A. G., Klein, P., and Ransil, B. J., *Epilepsia* 38:1082–1088, 1997; Catamenial epilepsy. Laidlaw, J. *The Lancet* 271:1235, 1956; Catamenial epilepsy: a review. Newmark, M. E., and Penry, J. K. *Epilepsia* 21:281, 1980; Medroxyprogesterone treatment of women with uncontrolled seizures. Mattson, R. H., Klein, P. E., Caldwell, B. V., et al. *Epilepsia* 23:436, 1982; Progesterone therapy in women with complex partial and secondary generalized seizures. Herzog A. G. *Neurology* 45:1660–1662, 1995; Ovulatory function in epilepsy. Cummings, L. N., Giudice, L., and Morrell, M. J. *Epilepsia* 36:355–359, 1995; Menstruation-related periodic hypersomnia: a case study with successful treatment. Sachs, C., Persson, H. E., and Hagenfeldt, K. *Neurology* 32:1376, 1982; Chronic recurrence of spontaneous pneumothorax due to endometriosis of the diaphragm. *JAMA* 168:2013, 1958; Catamenial pneumothorax. Lillington, G. A., and Mitchell, S. P. *JAMA* 219:1328, 1972; Spontaneous pneumothorax: a retrospective review of 210 consecutive admissions to Royal Perth Hospital. Watt, A. G. *Med. J. Aust.* 1:186, 1978; Catamenial pneumothorax—a literature review and report of an unusual case. Schoenfeld, A., Ziv, E., Zeelel, Y., et al. *Ob. Gyn. Surv.* 41:20, 1986; Recurring spontaneous pneumothorax associated with menstruation. Crutcher, R. R., Waltuch,

T. L., and Blue, M. E. *J. Thorac. Cardiovasc. Surg.* 54:599, 1967; Postcoital catamenial pneumothorax. Report of a case not associated with endometriosis and successfully treated with tubal ligation. Muller, N., and Nelms, B. *Am. Rev. Respir. Dis.* 134:803, 1986; Endometriosis within the thorax: Metaplasia, implantation or metastasis? Yeh, T. J. *Thorac. Cardiovasc. Surg.* 53:201, 1967; A clinical and pathologic study of endometriosis of the lung. Lattes, R., Shepard, F., Tovell, H., et al. *Surg. Gynec. Obstet.* 103:552, 1956; A cure for pneumothorax during menstruation. Eckford, S. D., and Westgate, J. *The Lancet* 347:734, 1996; Endometriosis and infertility. In *Modern Approaches to Endometriosis.* Rock Jr., T. E., ed. Kluwer Academic Publishers, Dordrecht, 1991; Peritoneal endometriosis due to menstrual dissemination of endometrial tissue in the peritoneal cavity. Sampson, J. A. *Am. J. Obstet. Gynecol.* 14:422–469, 1927; Pelvic pain and endometriosis. Maclaverty, C. M., and Shaw, R. W. In *Endometriosis. Current Understanding and Management.* Shaw, R. W., ed. Blackwall Science, Oxford, 1995; The distribution of endometriosis in the pelvis by age groups and infertility. Redwine, D. B. *Fertil. Steril.* 47:173–175, 1987; Induced amenorrhea in the prevention of endometriosis: a proposal for the third millennium. Coutinho, E. M. In *Progress in the Management of Endometriosis.* Coutinho, E. M., Spinola, P., and de Moura, L., eds. Parthenon, London and New York, 1995; *Marilyn Monroe: The Biography.* Spoto, D. HarperCollins, New York, 1993; *Goddess: The Secret Lives of Marilyn Monroe.* Summers, A. Onyx, Penguin Books, 1986; Regression of uterine leiomyomas after treatment with gestrinone, an anti-estrogen, anti-progesterone. Coutinho, E. M., Azadian-Boulanger, G., and Goncalves, M. T. *Am. J. Obstet. Gynecol.* 155:761–767, 1986; Thyroid function and treatment in premenstrual syndrome. Nicolai, T. F., Mulligan, G. M., and Gribble, R. K. *J. Clin. Endocrinol. & Metabol.* 70:1108, 1990; Recurrent herpes labialis, recurrent ulcers and the menstrual cycle. Segal, A. L., Katcher, A. H., Brightman, V. J., et al. *J. Dent. Res.* 53:797, 1974; Incidence of recurrent herpes labialis and upper respiratory infection: a prospective study of the influence of biologic, social and psychologic predictors. Friedman, E., Katcher, A. H., and Brightman, V. J. *Oral Surg. Oral Med. Pathol.* 43:873, 1977; The causation of appendicitis. Short, A. R. *Br. J. Surg.* 8:171, 1920; Acute appendicitis risk in various phases of the menstrual cycle. Arnbjornsson, E. *Acta. Chir. Scand.* 149:603, 1983; *Anemia through the Ages: Changing Perspectives and Their Implications in Diet, Demography and Disease.* Kent, S., Stuart-Macadam, P., and Kent, S., eds. Aldine de Gruyter, New York, 1992; Iron deficiency and other acquired anemias. Kent, S. In *The Cambridge Historical Geographical and Cultural Encyclopedia of Human Nutrition.* Kipple, K. ed. Cambridge University Press, Cambridge, 1992; The liabilities of iron deficiency. Cook, J., and Lynch, S. *Blood* 68:803–809, 1986; Iron deficiency. Scrimshaw, N. *Sci. Am.* 265:46–52, 1991; Iron. Kent, S., and Stuart-Macadam, P. In *The Cambridge Historical Geographical and Cultural Encyclopedia of Human Nutrition.* Kipple, K. ed. Cambridge University Press, Cambridge, 1992; Physiological, pathological and dietary influences on the hemoglobin level. Wadsworth, G. R. In *Diet, Demography and Disease.* Stuart-Macadam, P., and Kent, S., eds. Aldine de Gruyter, New York, 1992; Determination of menstrual blood loss. Holberg, L., and Nilsson, L. *Scand. J. Clin. Lab. Invest.* 16:244–248, 1964; The blood loss during normal menstruation. Barer, A. P., and Fowler, W. M. *Am. J. Obstet. Gynecol.* 31:979–986, 1936; Iron metabolism in normal young women during consecutive menstrual cycles. Leverton, R. M., and Roberts, W. M. *J. Nutr.* 13:65–71, 1937; Consequences of uterine blood loss caused by various intrauterine devices in South American women. Andrade, A. T. L., Pizarro, E., Shaw, S. T., Souza, J. P., Belsey, E. M., and Rowe, P. *Contraception* 38:1–18, 1988; Intrauterine contraception with copper T device. Hagenfeldt, K. *Contraception* 6:37–54, 1972; Menstrual blood loss in iron deficiency anemia. Jacobs, A., and Butler, E. B. *The Lancet* 2:407–409, 1965; Fever and reduced iron. Their interaction as host defense to bacterial infection. Kluger, M., and Rottenburg, B. *Science* 203:374–376, 1979; Iron and risk of cancer. Stevens, R. *Medical Oncology and Tumor Pharmacotherapy* 72(⅔):177–181, 1990; Blood letting, iron hemeostasis and human health. Weinberg, R. J., Ell, S. R., and Weinberg, E. D. *Medical Hypothesis* 21:441–443, 1986; Iron-poor blood, iron-poor brain. *Health,* Time Publishing Ventures, Inc., San Francisco, September 1995; Randomized study of cognitive effects of iron supplementation in non-anemic, iron-deficient adolescent girls. Bruner, A. B., Joffe, A., Duggan, A. K., Casella, J. F., and Brandt, J. *The Lancet* 348:992–996, 1996.

CHAPTER 6: NATURAL SUPPRESSION OF MENSTRUATION

Menstruation during pregnancy. Yamanek, S. H. *The Lancet* 1:689, 1971; De la grossesse nerveuse a l'anorexie mentale. Demaret, A. *Acta Psychiatr. Belg.* 91:11–22, 1991; Case of the psychotherapeutic treatment of pseudo-pregnancy by pseudo-labor. Brankov, T. S. *Akushi. Ginekol.* (Sofia) 23:93–96, 1984; Herstellung von Pseudograviditäten bei Frauen durch hochdosierte der Frühgravidität angepaste hCG-Gaben. Geiger, W., Kaiser, R., and Kneer, M. *Acta Endocrinol.* (Copenhagen) 62:289–298, 1969; Pseudopregnancy induced by estrogen-progestogen alone in the treatment of endometriosis. Moghissi, K. S. *Prog. Clin. Biol. Res.* 323:221–232, 1990; Prolactin inhibits oestrogen synthesis in the ovary. Dorington, and J., and Gore Langton, R. E. *Nature* (London) 290:600–602, 1981; Physiological mechanisms underlying lactational amenorrhea. McNeilly, A. S., Tay, C. C., and Glasier, A. *Ann. NY Acad. Sci.* 709:145–155, 1994; *Reproductive Anthropology: Descent through Women.* Gebbie, D. A. M. John Wiley & Sons, New York, 1981; The evolution of endometrial cycles and menstruation. Strassmann; B. I. *Q. Rev. Biol.* 7(2):181–220, 1996; Predictors of fecundability and conception waits among the Dogon of Mali. Strassmann, B. I. et al. *Am. J. Phys. Anthropol.* 105(22):167–84, 1988; Population growth and the beginnings of sedentary life among the !Kung Bushmen. Lee, R. B. In *Population Growth: Anthropological Implications.* Spooner, B., ed., pp. 329–342. M.I.T. Press, Cambridge, MA, 1972; The population of the Dobe area !Kung. Howells, N. L. In *Kalahari Hunter Gatherers.* Lee, R. B., and De Yore, I., eds., pp. 137–151, Harvard University Press, Cambridge, MA, 1976; The female athlete. Wilkerson, L. A. *Am. Fam. Physician* 29:233–237, 1984; The relationship of exercise to anovulatory cycles in female athletes: hormonal and physical characteristics. Russel, J. B., Mitchell, D., Musey, P. L., and Collins, D. C. *Obstet. Gynecol.* 63:452–456, 1984; Delayed menarche in young women athletes. Ryan, A. J. *Ann. Hum. Biol.* 5:417–422, 1994; Age at menarche in athletes and non-athletes. Malina, R. M., Harper, A. B., Avent, H. H., and Cambbell, D. E. *Postgrad Med.* 67:52–53, 1980; Plasma corticotropin-releasing hormone, corticotropin and endorphins at rest and during exercise in eumenorrheic and amenorrheic athletes. Hoktari, H., Elovainio, R., Salminen, K., and Laatikainen, T. *Fertil. Steril.* 50:233–238, 1988; Menstrual dysfunction in Nigerian athletes. Toriola, A. L., and Mathur, D. N. *Br J Obstet. Gynaecol.* 93:979–985, 1986; Bone mineral content of amenorrheic and eumenorrheic athletes. Drinkwater, B. L., Nilson, K., Chestnut, C. H. III, Brumner, W. J., Shainholtz, S., and Southworth, M. B. *N. Engl. J. Med.* 311:277–281, 1984; Comparison of bone density in amenorrhoeic women due to athletics, weight loss and premature menopause. Jones, K. P., Ravnikar, V. A., Tulchinsky, D. and Schiff, I. *Obstet. Gynecol.* 66:5–8, 1985; High serum cortisol levels in exercise associated amenorrhea. Ding, J. H., Sheckter, C. B., Drinkwater, B. L., Soules, M. R., and Bremner, W. J. *Ann. Intern. Med.* 108:530–534, 1988; Are high-performance young women athletes doomed to become low-performance old wives? A reconsideration of the increased risk of osteoporosis in amenorrheic women. De Crue, C., Vermeulen, A., and Ostyn, M. *J. Sports Med. Phys. Fitness* 31:108–114, 1991; Spine and total body bone mineral density in amenorrheic endurance athletes. Rutherford, O. M. *J. Appl. Physiol.* 74:29004–29008, 1993; Bone mineral density and longterm exercise. An overview of cross-sectional athlete studies. Suominen, H. *Sports Med.* 16:316–330, 1993; Changes in bone mineral content in male athletes: mechanisms of action and intervention effects. Kleeges, R. C., Ward, K. D., and Shelton, M. L. *JAMA* 276:226–230, 1996; Gymnasts exhibit higher bone mass than runners despite similar prevalence of amenorrhea and oligomenorrhea. Robinson, T. L., Snow-Harter, C., Taaffe, D. R., Gillis, D., Shaw, J., and Marcus, R. *J. Bone Mineral Res.* 10:26–35, 1995; Bone density in women college athletes and older athletic women. Jacobsen, P. C., Beaver, W., Grubb, S. A., Taft, T. N., and Talmage, R. V. *J. Orthop. Res.* 2:328–332, 1985; Effects of resistance training on regional and total one mineral density in premenopausal women: a randomized prospective study. Lohman, T., Going, S., Pamenter, R., Hall, M., Boyden, T., Houtkooper, L., Ritenbaugh, C., Bare, L., Hill, A., and Aickin, M. *J. Bone Mineral Res.* 10:1015–1024, 1995; Menstrual dysfunction in swimmers: a distinct entity. Constantini, N. W., and Warren, M. P. *J. Clin. Endocrinol. Metab.* 80:2740–2744, 1995; Delayed menarche and amenorrhea of college athletes in relation to onset of training. Frisch, R. E., Gotz Welbergen, A. V., McArthur, J. W., Albright, T., Witschi, J., Bullen, B., Birnholz, J., Reed, R. B., and Hermann, H. *JAMA* 246:1559–1563, 1981; A physician survey of therapy for exercise-associated amenorrhea: a brief report. Haberland, C. A., Seddick, D., Marcus, R., Bachrach, L. K. *Clin. J. Sport Med.* 5:246–250, 1995; Menstrual dysfunction and hormonal status in athletic women: a review. Baker, E. R. *Fertil. Steril.* 36:691–696, 1981; Athletic activity and menstruation. Diddle, A. W. *South Med. J.* 76:619–624, 1983.

CHAPTER 7: MEDICAL SUPPRESSION OF MENSTRUATION

Hysterectomy in the United States 1965–1984. Pokras, R., and Hufnagel, V. G. *Am. J. Publ. Health* 78:852–861, 1988; Reassessing the hysterectomy. Lilford, R. J. *Orgyn* 4:6–10, Organon, Oss, The Netherlands, 1998; The hormonal causes of premenstrual tension. Frank, R. T. *Arch. Neur. Psych* 26:1053, 1931; Persistence of symptoms of premenstrual tension in hysterectomized women. Backstrom, C. T., Boyle, H., and Baird, D. T. *Br. J. Ob. Gyn* 88:530, 1981; *You Don't Need a Hysterectomy: New and Effective Ways of Avoiding Major Surgery.* Strausz, I. K. Addison-Wesley, Publishing Co., New York, 1994; *The No-Hysterectomy Option.* Goldfarb, H. A., and Greif, J. John Wiley & Sons, Inc., New York, 1990; Hysterectomy and autonomy. Bernal, E. W. *Theor. Med.* 9:73–81, 1988; The effect of hysterectomy on the age at ovarian failure: identification of a subgroup of women with premature loss of ovarian function and literature review. Saddle, N., et al. *Fertil. Steril.* 47:94–102, 1987; A post hysterectomy syndrome. Richards, D. H. *The Lancet* 2:983, 1974; Hysteroscopic endometrial ablation: using the rollerball electrode. Daniell, J. F. *Obstet. Gynecol.* 80:329–333, 1992; Premenstrual syndrome improvement after laser ablation of the endometrium for menorrhagia. Lefler, H. T. *J. Reprod. Med.* 34(11): 905, 1989; Transcervical resection of endometrium in women with menorrhagia. Magos, A. L., Baumann, R., and Turnbull, A. C. *Br. Med. J.* 298:1209–1212, 1989; Dragging technique versus blanching technique for endometrial ablation with Nd: YAG laser in the treatment of chronic menorrhagia. Lomano, J. M. *Am. J. Obstet. Gynecol.* 159:152–155, 1988; The effect of hysterectomy and bilateral oophorectomy in women with severe premenstrual syndrome. Casper, R. F., and Hearn, M. T. *Am. J. Obstet. Gynecol.* 162:105, 1990; Bilateral oopherectomy and hysterectomy in the treatment of intractable pelvic pain associated with pelvic congestion. Beard, W., et al. *Brit. J. Obstet. Gynaecol.* 98:988–991, 1991; Advances in the treatment of the premenstrual syndrome. Magos, A. *Br. J. Ob. Gynaecol.* 97:7–12, 1990; Lasting response to ovariectomy in severe intractable premenstrual syndrome. Casson, P., Hahn, P. M., and Van Nugt, D. A. *Am. J. Obstet. Gynecol.* 162: 99–105, 1990; A comparative study of intermittent versus continuous use of a contraceptive pill administered by vaginal route. Coutinho, E. M., O'Dwyer, E., Barbosa, I. C., Gu, Z. P., and Shaaban, M. M. *Contraception* 51:355, 1995; Conception control by monthly injections of medroxyprogesterone suspension and a long acting estrogen. Coutinho, E. M., and de Souza, J. C. *J. Reprod. Fertil.* 15:209–214, 1968; Induced amenorrhea in the prevention of endometriosis: a proposal for the third millennium. Coutinho, E. M. In *Progress in the Management of Endometriosis.* Coutinho, E. M., Spinola, P., and de Mara, L., eds. Parthenon, London and New York, 1995; Conservative treatment of uterine leiomyomas with the antiestrogen, antiprogesterone, R-2323. Coutinho, E. M. *Int. J. Gynecol. Obstet.* 19:357, 1981; Influence of the LH-RH analogue buserelin on cycle ovarian function and the endometrium: a new approach to fertility control? Schmidt-Gollwitzer, M., Hardt, W., and Schmidt-Gollwitzer, K. *Contraception* 23:187–196, 1981; Inhibition of ovulation in women by intranasal treatment with luteinizing hormone-releasing hormone agonist. Bergquist, C., Nillius, S. J., and Wide, L. *Contraception* 19:497–506, 1979; Clinical experience with implant contraception. Coutinho, E. M. *Contraception* 18:411–427, 1978; Contraception with long-acting subdermal implants: a five year clinical trial with silastic covered rod implants containing levonorgestrel. Robertson, D. L., Diaz, S., Alvarez-Sanchez, F., Mishell, D., Coutinho, E. M., et al. *Contraception* 31:4:351, 1985; Multicenter clinical trial on the efficacy and acceptability of a single contraceptive implant of nomegestrol acetate, Uniplant. Coutinho, E. M., de Souza, J. C., Athayde, C., Barbosa, I. C., Alvarez, F., Brache, V., Gu, Z. P., Emuveyan, E. E., Adekunle, A. O., Devoto, L., Shaaban, M. M., Salem, H. T., Affandi, B. Acosta, O. M., Mati, J., and Ladipo, O. A. *Contraception* 53:121–125, 1996; A 4-year pilot study on the efficacy and safety of Implanon®. Kiriwat, A., and Coelingh Bennink, H. J. T. *European Journal of Contraception and Reproductive Health Care* 3:85–91, 1998; ST-1435: a new alternative for medical therapy of endometriosis. Coutinho, E., Carreira, C., and Bastos, G. J. O. In *Progress in the Management of Endometriosis.* Coutinho, E. M., Spinola, P., and de Moura, L. H., eds, pp. 333–336. Parthenon Publishing, U.K., 1995; Contraceptive effectiveness of silastic implants containing the progestin R-2323. Coutinho, E. M., da Silva, A. R., Carreira, C. M., Chaves, M. C., and Adeodato Filho, J. *Contraception* 11:625–635, 1975; Cardiovascular disease and steroid hormone contraceptives. Report of a scientific group. Geneva, The World

Health Organization, 1998 (WHO technical report series, No.877); Hormone replacement therapy and heart disease prevention. Petitti, D. *JAMA* 280:650–651, 1998; The reduction in risk of ovarian cancer associated with oral contraceptive use. Centers for Disease Control and the NICHD. *N. Engl. J. Med.* 316:650–655, 1987; "Incessant ovulation" and ovarian cancer. Casagrande, J. T., Pike, M. C., Ross, T. K., Louie, E. W., Roy, S., and Henderson, B. E. *The Lancet* 170–173, July 1979; Menopausal hormone replacement therapy and breast cancer: a meta-analysis. Sillero-Anemas, M. et al. *Obstet. Gynecol.* 79(2):286–294, 1992; Effects of chronic sulpiride induced hyperprolactinemia on menstrual cycle of normal women. Oseko, F., Morikava, K., Motohashi, T., and Aso, T. *Obstet. Gynecol.* 72: 267–270, 1988; Alternatives to conventional hormone replacement. Taylor, M. *Menopausal Medicine* 6:1–6, 1998; Trends in alternative medicine use in the United States, 1990–1997. Eisenberg, D. M., et al. *JAMA* 280(18):1569–1575, 1998.

CHAPTER 8: IN SUPPORT OF MENSTRUATION
Juice of Life: The Symbols and Magic Significance of Blood. Camporesi, P. Continuum Publishing Company, New York, 1995; *Blood Magic: The Anthropology of Menstruation.* Buckley, T., and Gottlieb, A., eds. University of California Press, Los Angeles, 1988; Menstruation: an ethnophysiological defense against pathogens. Sobo, E. J. *Perspectives in Biol. & Med.* 38:36–39, 1994; *Menstrual Health in Women's Lives.* Dan, A. J., and Lewis, L. L., eds. University of Illinois Press, Urbana and Chicago, 1992. *The Curse: A Cultural History of Menstruation.* Delaney, J., Lupton, M. J., and Toth, E. University of Illinois Press, Urbana and Chicago. 1988; Menopause and coronary heart disease. Gordon, T., Kannel, M. C., Hjortland, C., and McNamara, P. M. *Annals of Internal Medicine* 89:157–161, 1978; The effects of estradiol on blood lipids and lipoproteins in postmenopausal women. Fahraeus, L. *Obstet. & Gynecol.* 72:188–228, 1988; Quality of life issues in the management of the menopause. Speroff, L. In *Women's Health Today.* Popkin, D., and Peddle, L., eds. Parthenon, New York, 1994; Hormone replacement therapy reduces the reactivity of monocytes and platelets in whole blood—A beneficial effect on artherogenesis and thrombus formation? Aune, B., Oian, P., Omsjo, I., and Osterud, B. *Am. J. Obstet. Gynecol.* 173:1816–1825, 1965; The effect of estrogen replacement therapy with or without progestogen on the fibrinolytic system and coagulation inhibitors in post menopausal status. Gilabert, J., Estelles, A., Cano, A., Espana, F., Barrachina, R., Grancha, S., Aznar, J., and Tortajada, M. *Am. J. Obstet. Gynecol.* 173:1849–1854, 1995; Menopause, hormone replacement therapy and cardiovascular disease: a review of haemostaseological findings. Winkler, V. H. *Fibrinolysis* 6 (suppl. 3):5–10, 1992; Iron and the sex difference in heart disease risk. Sullivan, J. L. *The Lancet* 1:1293–1294, 1981; The iron paradigm of ische-

mic heart disease. Sullivan, J. L. *Am. Heart J.* 117:1177–1188, 1989; Post-menopausal use of estrogen and occlusion of coronary arteries. Gruchow, H. W., Anderson, A. J., and Barboriak, J. J. *Am. Heart J.* 115:954, 1988; Overview of the efficacy of hormonal replacement therapy. Ettinger, B. *Am. J. Obstet. Gynecol.* 165:1298–1301, 1987; Effects of estrogen replacement therapy on serum lipid values and angiographically defined coronary artery disease in postmenopausal women. Hong, M. K., Romm, P. A., and Reagan, K. *Am. J. Cardiol.* 69:176, 1992; Starvation infection: suppression and refeeding activation of an ecological necessity? Murray, M. J., and Murray, A. B. *The Lancet* 1:123–125, 1977; *Lectures on Clinical Medicine.* Trousseau, A., Bazine, P. V., et al. 5 vol. London, 1868–1872; *Symposium of Tuberculosis.* Heaf, F. R. G. London, 1957; In defense of ancient bloodletting. Brain, P. *S. Afr. Med. J.* 56:149–154, 1979; Immunity, transferrin and survival in Kwashiorkor. McFarlane, H., Reddy, S., Adcock, K. J., Adeshina, H., Cooke, A. R., and Akene, J. *Brit. Med. J.* 4:268–270, 1970; Somali food shelters in the Ogaden famine and their impact on health. Murray, M. J., Murray, A. B., Murray, M. B., and Murray, C. J. *The Lancet* 1:1283–1285, 1976; Food intake and resistance to disease. Mann, G. V. *The Lancet* 1:1238–1239, 1980; A prospective study of plasma ferritin and risk of myocardial infarction in U.S. physicians. Stampfer, M. J., Grodstein, F., Rosenberg, I., Willet, W., and Hemekens, C. *Circulation* 87:688, 1993; Low iron binding capacity as a risk factor for myocardial infarction. Magnusson, M. K., Sigfusson, N., Sigvaldason, H., Johanneson, G. M., Magnusson, S., and Thorgeirsson, G. *Circulation* 89:102–108, 1994; Iron and susceptibility to infectious disease. Weinberg, E. D. *Science* 184:952–956, 1974; Iron withholding in prevention of disease. In *Diet, Demography and Disease.* Weinberg, E. D., Stuart-Macadam, P., and Kent, S., eds. Aldine de Gruyter, New York, 1992; Premenopausal hysterectomy and cardiovascular disease. Centerwall, B. S. *Am. J. Obstet. Gynecol.* 139:58–61, 1981; Age at menopause as a risk factor for cardiovascular mortality. Van der Shouw, Y. T., Van der Graaf, Y., Steyerberg, E. W., Eijkemans, M. J. C., and Banga, J. D. *The Lancet* 347:714, 1996; The protective role of progesterone in the prevention of endometrial cancer. Greenblatt, R. B., Gambrell, R. D. Jr., and Stoddart, L. D. *Path. Res. Pract.* 174:297–302, 1982; Menstruation as a defense against pathogens transported by sperm. Profet, M. *Quarterly Rev. Biol.* 68:335–381, 1993; Sexist diseases. Garennee, M., and Lafon, M. *Perspectives in Biol. & Med.* 41:176–189, 1998; Timing of sexual intercourse in relation to ovulation. Effects on the probability of conception, survival of the pregnancy and sex of the baby. Wilcox, A. J., Weinberg, C. R., and Baird, D. D. *N. Engl. J. Med.* 333:1517–1521, 1995; Contraception and the etiology of pelvic inflammatory disease: new perspectives. Senanayake, P., and Kramer, D. G. *Am. J. Obstet. Gynecol.* 138:852–859, 1980; The protective influence of progestagen only contraception against vaginal moniliasis. Toppozada, M. *Contraception* 20:99–102, 1979; The evolution of endometrial cycles and menstruation. Strassmann, B. I. *Quarterly Rev. Biol.* 71:181–218, 1996; Contraception and toxic shock syndrome: a reanalysis. Shelton, J. D., and Higgins, J. E. *Contraception* 24:631–636, 1981.

CHAPTER 9: ABSENCE OF MENSTRUATION AND DISEASE
The syndrome of androgen resistance. Griffin, J. E., and Wilson, J. D. *N. Engl. J. Med.* 302:198–209, 1980; Male pseudohermaphroditism consistent with 17–20 desmolase deficiency. Goebelsmann, V., Zachmann, M., Davajan, V., Israel, R., Westman, J. H., and Mishell, D. R. *Gynecol. Obstet. Invest.* 7:138–156, 1976; Pediatric and adolescent gynecology. Muran, D. In *Current Obstetric and Gynecologic Diagnosis and Treatment.* Delherney, A. H., and Pernoll, M. L., eds. 8th ed. Prentice-Hall International, Appleton & Lange, CT, 1994; Mumps oophorits, a cause of premature menopause. Morrison, J. C., Givens, J. R., Wiser, W. L., and Fish, A. S. *Fertil. Steril.* 26:655, 1975; Chromosomal and clinical findings in 110 females with Turner's syndrome. Palmer, C. G., and Reichman, A. *Human Genet.* 34:35–43, 1976; Gonadal anomalies and dysgenesis. In *Progress in Infertility.* Morris, J., Behrman, S. J., and Kistner, R. W., eds. Little, Brown, Boston, 265–279, 1975; Premature ovarian failure. Aiman, J., and Smentek, C. *Obstet. Gynecol.* 66:9–14, 1985; Idiopathic premature ovarian failure: clinical and endocrine characteristics. Rebar, R. W., Krickson, G. F., and Yen S. S. C. *Fertil. Steril.* 37:35–41, 1982; Post-partum necrosis of the anterior pituitary. Sheehan, H. L. *J. Path. & Bact.* 45:189–214, 1937; Endocrine function after spontaneous infarction of the human pituitary: report review and reappraisal. Veldhuis, J. D., and Hammond, J. M. *Endocr. Rev.* 1:100–107, 1980; Empty sella: review of 76 cases. Jaffer, K. A., Obbens, E. A., and El Gamal, T. A. *South Med. J.* 72:294–296, 1979; Pituitary tumors: diagnosis and management. Molitch, M. E. *Endocrinol. Metab. Clin. North Am.* 16:503–528, 1987; Management of prolactinomas. Molitch, M. E. *Ann. Rev. Med.* 40:225–232, 1989; Galactorrhea: 235 cases including 48 with pituitary tumors. Kleinberg, D. L., Noel, G. L., and Frantz, A. G. *N. Engl. J. Med.* 296:589–600, 1977; Current concepts and treatment of hyperprolactinemia. Archer, D. F. *Obst. Gynecol. Clin. North Am.* 14:979–998, 1987; Vaginal administration of bromocriptine to treat inappropriate hyperprolactinemia. Spinola, P. G., Coutinho, E. M., Barbosa, I. C., and Vianna, S. *Archives of Gynecology* 237 (suppl.):299, 1985; Pituitary micro adenomas causing Cushing's disease respond to corticotropin-releasing factor. Orth, D. N., Debold, C. R., De Chemey, G. S., et al. *J. Clin. Endocrinol. Metab.* 55:1017, 1982; *The Nobel Duel.* Wade, N. Anchor Press, Doubleday, New York, 1981; Hypothalamic dysfunction in patients with anorexia nervosa. Mecklenburg, R. S., Loriaux, D. L., Thompson, R. H., Andersen, A. K., and Lipsett,

M. B. *Medicine* 53:147–159, 1974; Anorexia nervosa: behavioral and hypothalamic aspects. Vigersky, R. A., Poriaux, D. L., Andersen, A. K., and Lipsett, M. B. *J. Clin. Endocrinol. Metab.* 5:517–535, 1976; Anorexia nervosa and bulimia. Warren, M. P. In *Gynecology and Obstetrics*, ed. Sciarra, J. J. Harper & Row, NJ, vol. 5, chapter 26, 1988; The endocrinology of anorexia nervosa. Walsh, B. T. *Psychiatr. Clin. North Am.* 3: 299–319, 1980; LHRH: clinical applications growing. Ziporeyn, T. *JAMA* 253:469–476, 1985; Hypercortisolism in patients with functional and hypothalamic amenorrhea. Suh, B. Y., Liu, J. H., Berga, S. L., Quigley, M. E., Laughlin, G. A., and Yeu, S. S. *J. Clin. Endocrinol. Metab.* 66:733–739, 1988; Weight loss in secondary amenorrhea. Homberg, N. G., and Nylander, I. *Acta Obstet. Gynecol. Scand.* 50:241–246, 1971; Amenorrhea secondary to voluntary weight loss. Graham, R. L., Grimes, D. L., and Gambrele, R. D., Jr. *South Med. J.* 72:1259–1261, 1979; The influence of dieting on the menstrual cycle of healthy young women. Pirke, K. M., Schweiger, V., Lemmel, W., Krieg, J. C., and Berger, M. *J. Clin. Endocrinol. Metab.* 60:1174–1179, 1985; Kallmann, F., Schonfield, W. A., and Barrera, S. E. *Am. J. Mental Defic.* 48:203–236, 1944; Chemical induction of ovulation. Greenblatt, R. B. *Fertil. Steril.* 12:402, 1961; Duration of infertility following ovarian wedge resection. Stein, I. F. *West. J. Surg.* 72:237–240, 1964.

Index